CANCER PAIN

This book is dedicated to patients with cancer pain. The editors will devote their royalty payments to provide free copies for doctors in the developing countries of the world.

CANCER PAIN

Edited by

MARK SWERDLOW

Honorary Consultant, Regional Pain Relief Centre,
Hope Hospital, University of Manchester School
of Medicine, Eccles Old Road, Salford M6 8HD, UK

and

VITTORIO VENTAFRIDDA

Director, Division of Pain Therapy, National
Cancer Institute, Via Venezian 1, 20133 Milan, Italy

Director, WHO Collaborating Centre for Cancer
Pain Relief, Milan, Italy

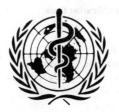

The expression of opinions herein does not necessarily represent the
decisions or the stated policy of the World Health Organization.

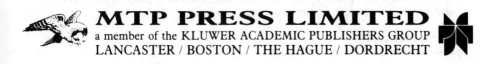

MTP PRESS LIMITED
a member of the KLUWER ACADEMIC PUBLISHERS GROUP
LANCASTER / BOSTON / THE HAGUE / DORDRECHT

Published in the UK and Europe by
MTP Press Limited
Falcon House
Lancaster, England

British Library Cataloguing in Publication Data

Cancer pain.

    1. Cancer—Palliative treatment
    2. Analgesia
    I. Swerdlow, Mark   II. Ventafridda, Vittorio
    616'.99'4   RC270.8

    ISBN 0–85200–858–9
    ISBN 0–85200–990–9 Pbk

Published in the USA by
MTP Press
A division of Kluwer Academic Publishers
101 Philip Drive
Norwell, MA 02061, USA

Library of Congress Cataloging in Publication Data

Cancer Pain.

    Includes bibliographies and index.
    1. Cancer—Complications and sequelae. 2. Intractable
Pain. 3. Analgesia. I. Swerdlow, Mark. II. Ventafridda
Vittorio. [DNLM: 1. Neoplasms. 2. Pain—therapy.
QZ 200 C2153633]
RC262.C29118   1986   616.99'4   86–20994

    ISBN 0–85200–858–9
    ISBN 0 85200–990–0 (pbk.)

Typeset and printed by
Butler & Tanner Ltd, Frome and London

Contents

List of Contributors

Sven Andersson
Department of Physiology
University of Goteborg
PO Box 33031,
S-400 33 Goteborg,
Sweden

Alberto Azzarelli
Division of Clinical
Oncology 'G',
National Cancer Institute,
Via Venezian 1,
20133 Milan,
Italy

Mary Baines
Consultant Physician,
St. Christopher's Hospice,
51–53 Lawrie Park Road,
Sydenham,
London SE26 6DZ,
United Kingdom

Michael R. Bond
Department of Psychological
    Medicine,
University of Glasgow,
6 Whittinghame Gardens,
Great Western Road,
Glasgow G12 0AA,
United Kingdom

John J. Bonica
Chairman Emeritus and
    Professor,
School of Medicine,
Department of Anesthesiology
    RN–10,
University of Washington,
Seattle, Washington 98195,
USA

Sergeo Crispino
Division of Oncology,
National Cancer Institute,
Via Venezian 1,
20133 Milan,
Italy

Kathleen M. Foley
Chief,
Pain Service,
Memorial Sloan–Kettering
  Cancer Center,
1275 York Avenue,
New York NY 10021,
USA

Edward R. Hitchcock
Professor of Neurosurgery and
  Neurology,
Midland Centre for Neuro-
  surgery and Neurology,
Holly Lane,
Smethwick,
Warley,
West Midlands B67 7JX,
United Kingdom

Silvio Monfardini
Scientific Director,
Cancer Institute,
33081 Aviano (Pordenone),
Italy

Alberto Scanni
Division of Oncology,
Ospedale Fatabene Fratelli,
Milan,
Italy

Mark Swerdlow
Honorary Consultant,
Regional Pain Relief Centre,
Hope Hospital,
University of Manchester School
  of Medicine,
Eccles Old Road,
Salford M6 8HD,
United Kingdom

Robert G. Twycross
Consultant Physician,
Sir Michael Sobell House,
The Churchill Hospital,
Headington,
Oxford,
United Kingdom

Vittorio Ventafridda
Director,
Division of Pain Therapy,
National Cancer Institute,
World Health Organization
  Collaborating Centre for
  Cancer Pain Relief,
Via Venezian 1,
20133 Milan,
Italy

Foreword

When the editors asked me to write a foreword to this book I felt very honoured but somewhat embarrassed. I am not a physician but I have spent many years dealing with the organizational problems of the care and assistance of cancer patients who have no hope of recovering.

The Floriani Foundation became active in 1977 with a donation from my wife and myself following a sad family experience. The aim of this Foundation is to assist research, studies and diffusion of information in order to better the quality of life of people suffering from debilitating chronic disease, the most important of which is cancer. In the past the Floriani Foundation has sponsored and organized congresses and meetings on the subject of cancer pain relief. The proceedings of those meetings were published and have reached a limited number of people, mainly specialists in this field.

It is therefore a pleasure to have been able to help the editors of this book which should reach a much wider audience, particularly among those general practitioners in the developed and developing countries who are directly involved in the treatment of these suffering populations. I hope that the information it contains will be useful in offering support to these suffering patients who still receive very little attention from medical practice.

Many people prefer to die at home and their family doctor must have the knowledge and the means of supporting them medically through the trying last months of life, just as the community must organize to comfort and support them socially and psychologically at this time. Doctors in the more remote countries of the world and even those in peripheral parts of more medically advanced countries may have little access to information about the best methods of providing relief for cancer pain. It is with pleasure that I commend this book which will provide them with that information.

VIRGILIO FLORIANI

Preface

Many, but not all, patients with cancer suffer pain, particularly in the later stages of the disease. In recent years a great deal has been learned about the causes of this pain and about effective methods of relieving it. However, even in the more medically advanced countries of the world, where both methods and knowledge are available, cancer pain is not always satisfactorily dealt with. Many of the developing countries at present have neither adequate agents or knowledge.

The World Health Organization has published a handbook *Cancer Pain Relief* which presents the first international consensus on the subject of relief of cancer pain by drug therapy. Drugs are the mainstay of cancer pain treatment and properly used will effectively relieve 80–90% of cases. The present editors were involved in the preparation of the WHO handbook.

The purpose of the present book is to complement WHO *Cancer Pain Relief* by providing an account of the other modalities – oncological, nerve blocking, neurosurgical – which may help the other 10–20% of patients as well as providing information on terminal care and the care of symptoms other than pain. The present book provides an explanation of the rationale behind the use of each type of treatment, the technical details of the procedures, indications for use, the likely side-effects, selection of patients and selection of techniques.

There already exists a number of books on the treatment of chronic pain and of cancer pain in particular but they are in general too expensive and too technical to meet the needs of doctors working in rural areas and in the developing countries where, because of financial stringency, there may be limited equipment, drugs, staff and physical facilities.

The simpler measures, particularly drug treatment, should be available to every doctor and clinic in every country. For more specialized treatment the patient should be referred to the local hospital (i.e. the nearest hospital or health centre with surgery and/or oncological facilities).

We have tried to describe in detail all the methods and procedures for pain relief which could be applied by a family doctor or by doctors working in provincial non-teaching hospitals. More specialized techniques which are of value are only mentioned briefly but one or two references are given to authoritative works where further information on them could be obtained if needed. No attempt has been made to be academically comprehensive – methods which we consider to be of no real value or to be experimental have not been included.

We have tried to reach a reasonable compromise between the ideal and the practical. Thus, for example, in the absence of X-ray screening facilities, if paravertebral block would provide relief it is better to carry out a block 'blind' than not to do one at all. With regard to drugs, we have followed the WHO *Cancer Pain Relief* recommendations.

Continuity of care from hospital to home, from early pain management to management of the dying patient, should be available for all patients and should be an integral part of the management of their disease. We must stress that a purely technical approach may not be adequate; better results will always come from the combined care of motivated medical and paramedical staff plus family and friends.

We realize that conditions vary in different countries and the advice given here may need to be modified to suit local conditions.

Medical care is a continuum ranging from complete cure at one end to symptom control at the other. When cure is not possible anticancer palliation should be considered. When palliation is no longer possible, the emphasis moves to control of pain and other symptoms as an end in itself.

For a great majority of cancer patients pain relief may be the only realistic thing to offer.

The authors would be pleased to receive comments from doctors working in different parts of the world.

M.S.
V.V.

Acknowledgements

We are very grateful to Dr Kathleen Foley for considerable help at all stages of the preparation of this book. Without her help it might never have been written. We would also like to thank Dr J. Stjernswärd of the WHO Cancer Unit for his encouragement and support, and Dr Thelma Bates for her constructive comments.

The assistance given to us by the Floriani Foundation in the preparation of this book deserves our profound gratitude. We would also like to express our appreciation of the secretarial work carried out by Sigra Wanda Segre and Signa Miriam Vigotti.

A number of organizations have given their support to the publication of this book which has enabled it to be published at a modest cost and we would particularly like to acknowledge support from Dr Allan J. Miller of Napp Laboratories, Dr Corina Engler of Syntex Ltd and Dr Warwick Buckler of Boots Pharmaceuticals. Our thanks are also due to Dr J. R. Hall of Upjohn Ltd for providing most of the illustrations and to Professor D. Morley for help with the worldwide distribution.

The excellent indexing was carried out by Miss Patricia Cummings ALA to whom we are very grateful.

Finally, we must thank MTP Press (and particularly Mr P. Johnstone) for their cooperation at every stage of the preparation and printing of the book.

Acknowledgements

PART ONE
Basic Aspects of Cancer Pain

1

Importance of the Problem

J. J. Bonica

This book is devoted to a subject which is one of the most important and pressing issues of modern society – the effective control of cancer-related pain. Cancer-related pain afflicts millions of people worldwide every year. In addition to the severe psychological, emotional, affective, and economic impact of cancer pain in general, it has special attributes and significance to the patients and their families. All too frequently pain is inadequately managed and consequently many patients spend the last weeks, months or even years of their lives in great discomfort, suffering and disability which interfere with their quality of life.

This chapter is intended to emphasize the importance of cancer-related pain as a serious national and world health problem. The material will be presented in three sections, firstly the magnitude of the problem, including incidence and prevalence; then some important reasons for past deficiencies; and finally some recent trends and recommendations for future activities to improve this serious health problem.

MAGNITUDE OF THE PROBLEM

Pain is the most dreaded complication for the millions of people who develop cancer worldwide. Once the patients accept and adjust to the

3

news that they have cancer, one of the greatest problems is the fear of excruciating pain and suffering they believe will inevitably ensue.

In a survey of public opinion on cancer it has been found that pain ranked next to incurability in people's fear of cancer. It has also been found that the general public believes cancer to be much more painful than it actually is.

Overall prevalence of cancer pain

Moderate to severe pain is experienced by 30–45% of patients when cancer is diagnosed, by about 30–40% of the patients with intermediate stages of the disease, and by 60–100% of the patients with advanced or terminal cancer depending on the type and site of lesion. Careful analysis of the published reports also suggests (a) that in about 60–75% of cancer patients with pain it is moderate to severe in degree depending on the site and stage of the lesion, and (b) that most patients have two or more types of cancer-related pain syndromes (see page 38).

REASONS FOR THERAPEUTIC DEFICIENCIES

In view of the great advances in biomedical scientific knowledge and technology and especially the great amount of interest in, and effort devoted to, cancer research and therapy, why is cancer *pain* inadequately relieved?

Serious consideration of this important question suggests that it is due to an inadequate appreciation or outright neglect of the problem of pain (in contrast to the problem of cancer) by oncologists, medical educators, investigators, research institutions, and national and international cancer agencies. Consequently, there are great voids in our knowledge of various clinically relevant aspects of cancer pain, and whatever knowledge is currently available often is improperly applied.

Improper application of available knowledge and therapeutic modalities

The improper application of the knowledge and therapeutic modalities which are available is the most important reason for inadequate cancer pain relief because we have the drugs and other therapeutic modalities which, if properly applied, would provide good relief in most cancer patients. This sad state of affairs is not only the fault of the practising physician but must be shared by medical educators at the graduate and postgraduate levels. Review of the curricula of medical schools reveals that few, if any, teach students basic principles of the use of narcotics and other treatments that will effectively relieve cancer pain. Moreover, many physicians in residency training for specialization in surgical, medical and radiation oncology receive little or no teaching about the proper management of cancer pain. Usually the senior resident, who has vague and scanty information about cancer pain and its proper control, teaches the junior resident how to deal with the problem in a rather empirical way and passes on some of the misconceptions that will be mentioned below.

Inadequate or total lack of interest or concern about the problem of pain by oncologists is further shown by the fact that very little, if any, information about the proper management of the pain problem is found in the oncology literature.

As a result of this lack of education of students, graduate physicians, and other health professionals, the pain of cancer has been and continues to be treated in an empirical manner. Most practitioners rely on opioid analgesics. However, while they are very useful and have indeed a central role in the control of pain in cancer, they are often misused for a variety of reasons. In a small percentage of patients, potent opioids are used initially for mild pain which could be relieved by non-opioid analgesics alone or in combination with adjuvant drugs. At the other end of the spectrum of the problem, many, if not most, patients with moderate to severe pain of advanced cancer are given inadequate amounts of opioids or are given the right drug infrequently instead of at a regular interval. In all too many instances, physicians prescribe the analgesic but do not monitor the patient's response, or they fail to titrate the drug dose to the needs of the patient or fail to use adjuvant drugs when these are indicated.

The very high incidence of inadequate therapy of cancer pain with opioids is apparently due to insufficient knowledge of the pharmacology of these drugs and of the basic principles of managing cancer pain.

This problem of inadequate knowledge and misconception about the risk of addiction and opioid-induced depression is widespread. Apparently many physicians do not appreciate the fact that pain is a powerful respiratory stimulant and partially antagonizes the depressant effect of opioids. A physician can achieve good pain relief without hypoventilation by carefully titrating the drug administration to the needs of the patient. Moreover, there is impressive data that opioid addiction occurs rarely or not at all in patients receiving opioids for medical use even when administered for prolonged periods.

In patients with severe pain caused by recurrent or metastatic advanced cancer who are likely to require opioid therapy until death, addiction and physical dependence should not be considered as valid reasons for not giving opioids or for not giving them in adequate doses.

In some patients opioids and other systemic analgesics, even though properly administered, may not produce sufficient relief and other therapeutic modalities need to be used alone or in combination with these drugs. Unfortunately the role of these therapeutic modalities is not known by most practitioners and even by some oncologists. Consequently in most patients who could be more effectively relieved by a combination of these therapies, they are not considered or if they are considered they are applied too late. There is also a lack of personnel with interest and expertise in the proper application of these and other therapeutic modalities. Moreover, in some of these patients the cancer pain problem is such a complex array of sensory, perceptual, emotional and affective events that it requires the concerted and co-ordinated efforts of specialists from different disciplines working as a well co-ordinated team to achieve optimal results.

RECENT TRENDS AND THE FUTURE

Fortunately during the past decade or so a number of developments have taken place which if sustained and expanded hold the promise of helping to rectify some of the above deficiencies.

Some progress has been made in certain areas of pain diagnosis and therapy. An impressive number of physicians have manifested an interest in acquiring more knowledge about pain and its treatment as reflected in part by the large attendance at numerous postgraduate seminars, national meetings and world congresses. Another relatively recent encouraging trend has been the surge of interest in the multi-disciplinary approach to diagnosis and therapy of chronic pain and in the hospice concept of managing patients with terminal cancer.

In recent years there has also been some progress in regard to communication and diffusion of information. In addition to post-graduate courses there have been a number of national and inter-national symposia on cancer pain and a number of monographs and books containing relevant information have been published. There have been numerous international and national meetings to discuss the issues and problems in cancer pain management.

A most encouraging trend has been the activities of the Cancer Unit of WHO, which under the vigorous leadership of Dr Jan Stjernsward has developed a Cancer Pain Relief Program to improve the man-agement of patients with cancer worldwide. In 1982, the Unit initiated a preliminary survey of the prevalence of cancer pain in Brazil, India, Israel, Japan and Sri Lanka and the data acquired were presented at a workshop participated in by the editors of this volume and others who developed a methodology for the proper use of systemic analgesics and adjuvant drugs. These methods are being implemented in devel-oping countries worldwide.

Much needs to be done in the future if the millions of patients with cancer pain are to be managed effectively. This will require broadly-based multidisciplinary programmes in research, education, training and public information and also further improvement of patient care. This book should contribute significantly to the last issue for it will prove a highly effective source for the better understanding and treat-ment of cancer pain.

2

Neurophysiology and Biochemistry of Pain

S. Andersson

INTRODUCTION

Pain is experienced when a stimulus damages or threatens to damage the body tissue. In this respect, the sensation of pain is an important protective mechanism. A stimulus which causes pain – a 'noxious' stimulus – may also induce protective reactions such as withdrawal from the harmful object, and autonomic reactions such as changes in blood pressure, heart rate and respiration. Although certain behavioural aspects of the reaction to pain may be influenced by cultural factors, the reflex actions and the sensation elicited by a painful stimulus are physiological and are independent of learning.

Acute pain which occurs immediately on injury is often sharp (pinprick) and well localized. It may be followed later by a dull, aching or burning, ill-defined but unpleasant sensation similar to chronic pain. These two types of pain are attributed to different groups of afferent nerve fibres. *Acute* pain is mainly due to activity in thin myelinated fibres while *chronic* pain is primarily due to activity in unmyelinated fibres.

Pain reactions are associated with stimulation of *nociceptors*. These are special receptors which respond to painful stimuli. These receptors or their afferent nerves may also be activated and produce a sensation of pain during other conditions, e.g. inflammation in the tissue or

9

nerve compression. Such conditions may be longstanding and the pain becomes chronic.

In chronic pain the affected part of the body is immobilized and the pain is often dull and aching. Chronic pain can also arise without input from the peripheral nerves. In certain conditions pain seems to be due to changes within the central nervous system (CNS) itself. Such pain may occur after lesions of the peripheral nerves or in the CNS (e.g. thalamic pain after vascular lesions in the brain). In peripheral nerve lesions a longstanding noxious input may eventually change the connectivity in the central pain pathways so that even if the noxious input from the periphery is removed, the pain still persists due to the central changes.

The pain sensation following a given stimulus varies considerably in different situations. A soldier in combat may feel no pain after severe injuries whereas a similar damage would normally be very painful. The psychological state during the injury is of major importance to the appreciation of the pain intensity. Anxiety and fear for the future consequences of the injury causing the pain increase the suffering of the patient.

NEUROPHYSIOLOGICAL CHARACTERISTICS OF CANCER PAIN

Cancer pain is primarily produced by processes which affect nociceptors and their afferent peripheral nerve fibres. At present there are no indications that the pathophysiology of cancer pain is essentially different from that of other types of chronic pain. It is, however, possible that in certain conditions the cancer cells produce metabolites which have a potent action on nociceptors or afferent fibres, thus giving cancer pain a different dimension from other chronic pain.

Pain may arise from receptors and afferent fibres in the region of the primary tumour or its metastases or it may arise within the CNS due to the changed nervous activity produced by the impairment of function when cancer cells invade peripheral nerves. The primary cause of pain is often activation of receptors in various tissues (periosteum, ligaments, joints, skeletal muscles or visceral organs).

At first the afferent nerve fibres may be mechanically or chemically activated due to the invasion by cancer cells. At a later stage, the functional continuity of the nerve fibres can be interrupted causing degenerative processes in the remaining parts of the fibres. Their chemical content changes and 'sprouts' may form (see p. 12) and initiate pathological activity of similar type to that in a neuroma.

NOCICEPTORS

In most tissues and particularly in the skin there is a network of free nerve endings which are the terminals of thin nerve fibres. Many of these thin nerve fibres are activated by pain and temperature but some are excited by non-noxious mechanical stimuli.

Some receptors are associated with small myelinated (A-delta) primary afferents, others with unmyelinated (C) fibres. The *A-delta* afferents subserve mainly discriminative functions in nociception. Their discharge elicits the first, localized, sharp (pinprick) pain and may produce the withdrawal or flexion reflex. The *C-fibres* give rise to the aching and burning pain which is quite intolerable. This pain is not strictly localized; it is often referred to a large area even if the stimulus itself is localized.

The receptors of the slowly conducting C-fibres can be activated by high intensity mechanical, thermal or chemical stimulation and are thus 'polymodal' receptors. These receptors react to biochemical changes in the tissue. When the oxygen supply is inadequate, there will be accumulation of metabolites such as lactic acid and CO_2, the pH decreases and these nociceptors are activated. This may be the major cause of pain in conditions with inadequate arterial circulation such as angina pectoris and intermittent claudication.

The nature of the chemical activation is not fully understood: the effect may be mediated via algesic substances which are formed in the tissue and which modulate the excitability of nociceptors (e.g. prostaglandins, substance P and bradykinin). In cancer tumours the nociceptors may be influenced by the high metabolic activity in the cells. In addition, occlusion of blood vessels by the cancer may create ischaemia with a local decrease of pH and pO_2 and an increased accumulation of metabolic substances.

Inflammatory reactions with chemical changes may also lead to increased sensitivity of the nociceptors and, as a consequence, the nociceptors have a lower threshold to nociceptive stimuli.

Prostaglandins play an important role in the increased sensitivity of nociceptors after tissue damage and during inflammation. Prostaglandins are formed from arachidonic acid by the enzyme cyclooxygenase; they can be synthesized in almost every tissue of the body and each tissue produces different prostaglandins. Prostaglandins in small concentrations do not activate pain receptors. They can, however, potentiate the receptor sensibility to such an extent that normally non-noxious stimuli become painful. The increased sensitivity produced by prostaglandins is of considerable importance to the effect of bradykinin which facilitates the synthesis of prostaglandins. On the other hand, prostaglandin enhances the algogenic effect of bradykinin (Figure 1). The algogenic effect of prostaglandin can be counteracted by agents such as salicylates and indomethacin which inhibit the synthesis of prostaglandins.

In cancer pain mechanical stimulation of nociceptors occurs by increase in volume of encapsulated organs, by mechanical displacement of the tissue or by mechanical occlusion of hollow organs. The growing tumour may penetrate into organs and mechanically stimulate nociceptors. The mechanical stimuli affect receptors with increased sensitivity due to the chemical factors mentioned above.

Following nerve injury a burning pain may develop in the innervation territory of the affected nerve fibres. This pain can sometimes be relieved by surgical or chemical inactivation of the sympathetic innervation to the affected region, suggesting that the receptors are sensitive to noradrenaline. When a nerve is cut through, new fibres grow out of the proximal stump of the cut nerve; these 'sprouting' fibres are very sensitive to pressure, stretching or movement.

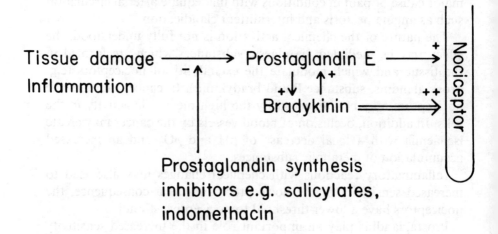

Figure 1 Prostaglandin action

REFLEX ACTIVATION OF NOCICEPTORS

Afferents from nociceptors have synaptic connections in the spinal cord with efferents to the skeletal muscles as well as to the sympathetic efferents (Figure 2). In certain conditions the nociceptive input may produce a positive 'feed-back loop' via the synaptic connections giving a self-sustained pain.

The sympathetic feed-back loop is particularly important during pain conditions in visceral organs (see p. 21). Noxious input from the gastrointestinal tract may increase the sympathetic tone leading to intestinal motor inhibition and decreased circulation. This effect can be lethal in conditions with ischaemia of the heart. The nociceptive activation increases the sympathetic tone causing a rise in heart rate and an increased oxygen demand.

The dorsal root

The cell bodies of all somatic afferent fibres are located in the dorsal root ganglia and the central portion of the neurons enter the spinal cord via the dorsal root. Small diameter fibres concentrate in the lateral portion of the rootlets.

However, a proportion (15–20%) of unmyelinated fibres do not go through the dorsal root but turn back from the dorsal root ganglion cells and enter the spinal cord via the ventral root. These fibres traverse the spinal cord and reach the dorsal part of the dorsal horn and

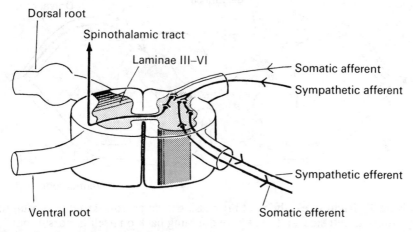

Figure 2   Synaptic connections

terminate in the same region as the unmyelinated fibres entering the cord via the dorsal root. This diversion of some unmyelinated fibres via the ventral root explains why dorsal rhizotomy does not always remove chronic pain (Figure 3).

Lesions of the dorsal root ganglia cells or the dorsal root fibres are followed by degeneration of the central part of the fibres. The nerve cells in the dorsal horn are deprived of input from the periphery. In this situation the discharge pattern of the cells in the pain pathway may change and they can be activated continuously giving rise to unremitting severe pain which is very difficult to relieve effectively ('deafferentation pain').

Dorsal horn mechanisms in nociception

After entering the dorsal spinal cord the C- and A-delta fibres branch and pass caudally or rostrally for up to three segments. Eventually the fibres terminate in the substantia gelatinosa (lamina I and II) of the dorsal horn which contains nociceptive cells (Figure 3). These cells respond only to noxious stimuli and the size of their receptive field is limited. The nociceptive input also reaches the deeper layers in the dorsal horn (lamina V) where the cells receive input from both low threshold and high threshold afferents. The cells may, for example, be activated by noxious stimuli in one peripheral area and by tactile

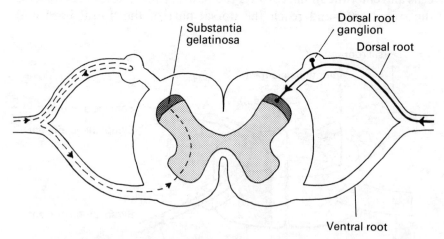

Figure 3   Right side – afferent fibre passing through dorsal root to substantia gelatinosa. Left side – afferent fibre doubling back on itself in dorsal root to re-enter cord via ventral root

stimuli in another area. The receptive field of these cells is often larger than that of nociceptive specific cells.

The region of termination of the C-fibres in the dorsal horn corresponds to the distribution of substance P and opiate bindings have also been demonstrated in the same area. The (superficially located) opiate receptor containing cells are activated pharmacologically by intrathecal injection of morphine. The morphine diffuses the short distance from the cord surface and binds to the opiate receptors in the inhibitory cells, which are activated.

Segmental inhibition of nociception is well known; it is due to collaterals from fibres ascending in the dorsal columns. It can be demonstrated by 'rubbing' or massaging an area. The mechanism is known as the 'Gate Control'. Large low threshold afferents from mechanoreceptors give off collaterals at the segmental level (Figure 2). Terminals for these collaterals excite interneurons which inhibit the transmission of impulses in nociceptive afferents and produce pain relief. The analgesic effect is strictly topographically arranged and effective pain relief can be obtained only by stimulation of low threshold receptors within the area of pain. Electrical stimulation of such receptors and their afferents is now being used to obtain complete or partial pain relief in certain chronic pain conditions. In cancer pain with nerve compression and decreased function in myelinated fibres the method is not effective.

Electrical stimulation of the dorsal columns of the cord via implanted electrodes has also been used to treat severe chronic pain. Dorsal column stimulation (DCS) may be effective in conditions with injuries of the peripheral nerves. The analgesic effect is due not only to antidromic activation of the segmental inhibitory mechanism but also to the involvement of nociceptive inhibitory systems at thalamic and cortical levels.

Descending inhibitory control

Several control systems descend from the brainstem to the spinal cord and control the transmission of nerve impulses from the nociceptive afferents to the relay cells in the dorsal horn.

Microinjection of morphine or electrical stimulation of the midbrain para-aqueductal grey matter (PAG) profoundly inhibits the neuronal responses in the spinal cord produced by noxious stimuli. Nerve fibres from PAG descend to the nucleus raphe magnus (Figure 4) which is one of the midline nuclei in the medulla oblongata. The cells in nucleus raphe magnus send their axons via the dorsolateral funiculus of the spinal cord to the segmental level. The fibres terminate in the substantia gelatinosa of the dorsal horn. The enkephalinergic nature of this descending system is clearly demonstrated by the reversal of its effect by administration of naloxone. This drug may inhibit the descending inhibition in PAG as well as in the spinal cord.

Administration of morphine systemically activates the endogenous opiate systems and thereby produces pain relief. Morphine exerts part of its action on opiate receptors in the brainstem. This effect can be demonstrated by local application of small amounts of the drug

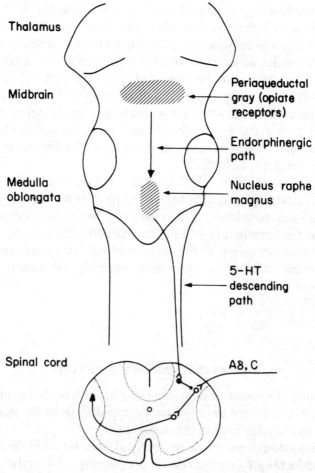

Figure 4 Midbrain and medulla

in PAG. The effective pain relief obtained by intrathecal morphine injection shows that activation of spinal opiate receptors also plays an important role in morphine analgesia. The analgesic effects of morphine can be reversed by the opiate antagonist naloxone.

The pain-controlling descending systems can be utilized to obtain relief of severe chronic pain. Electrical stimulation is given to nervous structures in the paraventricular region via electrodes implanted deep in the brain. The method is still in the experimental stage. Brain stimulation has been tested on patients with bilateral cancer pain and some patients are relieved. In these patients the stimulation has to be repeated several times a day. At present this method is used only in a few centres and it is not for routine treatment of pain.

The relation between muscle activity and increase in pain threshold may partly explain the finding that immobilized and inactive patients suffer more from pain than active patients. In pain conditions it is important to keep the patient mentally and physically active. A muscle training programme should be included in rehabilitation of pain patients.

Ascending pain pathways

The major ascending pain pathway is the *spinothalamic tract*. The nerve cells are situated in the dorsal horn and the axon crosses the midline to the opposite side and ascends to the thalamus (Figure 5). Transsection of this pathway has been used to control certain chronic pain conditions. The operation abolishes the pain and temperature sensations on the contralateral side of the body. The spinothalamic pathway consists of at least two divisions:

(1)   Cells in the dorsal horn receiving noxious input project to the specific somatosensory thalamic nucleus (VPL). This projection is somatotopically arranged and may subserve the discriminative component of pain.

(2)   A spinothalamic projection arises from cells in the dorsal horn with a similar spinal course but reaching the medial (intra-laminar) thalamic nuclei. This projection is characterized by pronounced convergence and the cells in the thalamus often receive excitation from the entire or large parts of the body. In addition to the noxious input, pathways from low threshold receptors also activate these cells. The medial projection system

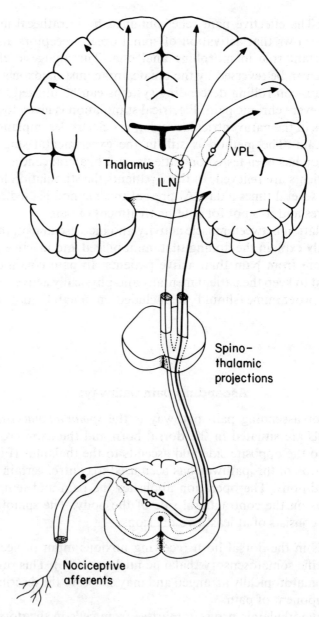

Figure 5 Spinothalamic tract

is less discriminative and may give rise to the pronounced aversive components in pain sensation.

In addition to the spinothalamic pathways nociceptive information also ascends elsewhere in the spinal cord. Following anterolateral cordotomy, pain may return after months or years. The responsible pathways are assumed to be multisynaptic consisting of long chains of neurons which project bilaterally to the brainstem reticular formation. It is interesting that the pain returning after anterolateral cordotomy is different and more difficult to accept than the original pain. This observation indicates that the nociceptive input reaches the consciousness via a route different from that in the intact subject.

The cerebral cortex

The cerebral cortex is considered to be of major importance in perception of sensory stimuli.

Little is known of the cortical mechanisms related to nociception. In fact, it has been questioned if the cortex is involved at all in the perception of pain. Electrical stimulation of the somatosensory cortex in conscious patients produces a sensation of tingling or numbness but not of pain. This suggests that the cortical neuronal systems in nociception are arranged differently from those mediating other sensations.

Clinically it is known that even extensive lesions in the cerebral cortex do not eliminate the pain sensation; indeed sometimes they may give rise to chronic pain.

Activity in low threshold afferent pathways inhibits the transmission from nociceptive pathways in cortical cells just as it does in the dorsal horn. Any stimulus co-activating nociceptors and low threshold afferents will inhibit the nociceptive input at several levels in the ascending system. In pain conditions with lesions of the large myelinated fibres, this inhibitory afferent system is not functioning adequately. Consequently, the nociceptive input caused by mechanical and chemical activation of nociceptive afferents is not balanced by inhibition and this may contribute to the production of pain.

Central changes related to cancer pain

As described previously chronic lesions of primary afferent fibres lead to changes in the afferent neuron and also to changes in the central structures innervated by these afferents. When cancer cells invade a peripheral nerve, changes in its central terminals are likely to occur. The dorsal horn cells normally receiving nociceptive input from the periphery may be denervated as are the inhibitory cells receiving input from low threshold afferents. The removal of inhibition may be an important factor in the production of persistent pain in cancer patients.

VISCERAL PAIN

In contrast to the skin there is no tactile sensibility in internal organs. Many types of receptor respond to physiological changes in the viscera or to mechanical distension but the main sensation from the internal organs that reaches the consciousness is that of pain. The physiological background of visceral pain receptors and their afferent connections is not completely known. Internal organs vary in pain sensitivity. Normally there are distensions and contractions (e.g. in intestine and gall bladder) without any conscious sensation. When distension and isometric contraction exceed a certain level, pain sensation appears. In pathological conditions, the sensibility of the receptors is markedly increased and stimuli which are normally non-noxious may produce severe pain.

Receptors signalling pain are situated in all layers of hollow organs. Visceral mechanoreceptors transmitting activity through C-fibres have been found in the smooth muscle layers in the wall of the small intestine, urethra and urinary bladder. The receptors are in series with muscle cells. These receptors respond by an increased activity to passive tension or active contraction in smooth muscle fibres. A strong increase in the activity occurs at isometric contraction as for example when the outlet from the gall bladder is obstructed. It has been assumed that the impulse flow in these fibres can give pain sensation only when their discharge frequency exceeds a certain level. Different receptor units show large fluctuations in threshold, probably due to varying tone in the smooth muscle fibres which are attached to them. Many visceral receptors fire at weak, non-noxious stimulation intensities and increase their discharge frequency markedly at intensities which are correlated with pain.

There is also evidence to suggest the existence of nociceptive specific visceral receptors. Such receptors have been found in the heart and respond to anoxia in the tissue. Other receptors respond to a high degree of mechanical distension, e.g. receptors in the gall bladder. They start to discharge at distension exceeding the physiological limit.

The enteric nervous system consists of a large number of cells intercalated between the receptors and the fibres projecting into the

CNS. The afferent pain fibres from visceral organs are found in the splanchnic, vagus and pelvic nerves. The large majority of fibres are thin, unmyelinated ones and terminate in the dorsal horn of the spinal cord or in the vagal nuclei. Most of the visceral afferents with cell bodies in the dorsal horn enter the spinal cord via the dorsal roots. About 20% of afferents reach the cord via the ventral roots. The presence of pain afferents in the ventral roots explains why pain may persist after dorsal rhizotomy. Pain from visceral afferents is often perceived as *referred pain*, that is with a false localization to a skin area in the appropriate dermatomes. The most probable explanation is that afferent fibres from viscera and skin converge towards the same neurons in the spinal cord and that the ascending axons from these cells are common for signals from skin and internal organs. The hypothesis of convergence also explains the hyperpathia and hyper-alagesia which may occur in a skin area due to activation of spinal neurons from visceral afferents.

The normal pain experienced on activation of an intact nervous system is different from that felt under pathological conditions when nerve signals are generated in an altered afferent system. Certain nerve fibres may be damaged or compressed, e.g. by a malignant growth, which may give similar changes in the perception of visceral pain as has been described with regard to somatic pain.

Recommended reading

1. Swerdlow, M. (ed.) (1986). *The Therapy of Pain*. 2nd Edn. (Lancaster: MTP Press).
2. Bonica, J.J. and Ventafridda, V. (eds.) (1979). *Advances in Pain Research and Therapy*. Vol. 2. (New York: Raven Press).

3

Psychological and Behavioural Aspects of Patient and Therapist

M. R. Bond

Most people fear the diagnosis of cancer, either because they have read or heard that it is almost always painful and fatal, or because they have personal experience of the drawn-out suffering of a close relative or friend, especially when treatment has been minimal or ineffectual.

The presence of pain is mentioned not only because it is greatly feared but also because it is known that its presence and increasing severity causes increasing levels of emotional distress.

EMOTIONAL DISORDERS IN CANCER PATIENTS

Cancer sufferers differ from others with chronic illness primarily because of the common view that the outcome will be death for most. From the outset, therefore, this colours the response of these patients to their illness. For example, the presence of early signs of cancer – weight loss or the presence of a mass, may be neglected out of ignorance or in some patients perhaps because of the fear that a diagnosis of cancer will be made. Almost all patients have moderate to severe anxiety from the moment an abnormality is detected and diagnosed.

23

In addition to anxiety, patients may experience feelings of help-lessness (because they are unable to influence the illness) and hope-lessness (if medical help seems inadequate). Both feelings are known to be associated with the development of depression. Worries also extend beyond the question of the physical effects of illness to concern about ability to work and the effects of the illness upon family life. The presence of pain and other disabling symptoms, including dyspnoea, vomiting and physical weakness, increase an individual's physical and social limitations and, as a consequence, his contact with friends. Also they mean increased dependence on other people and, therefore, a loss of personal freedom which, to some people, is a cause of great concern and unhappiness. Irritability and anger are also expressed by some cancer sufferers, partly as a result of feeling ill, and in particular because they often feel that life has been very unfair. Anger may be generated also because of a feeling that the control of the illness is inadequate.

The effects of treatment often add to the patient's discomfort and suffering. For example, the level of emotional distress and depression are increased by radiation and chemotherapy. Impairment of mental health is greatest with chemotherapy which produces very unpleasant side-effects, possibly lasting for some months after the cessation of treatment which, in itself, often occupies many weeks. The symptoms include lassitude, a mixture of depression and anxiety and sometimes there may be sexual difficulties. Physical mutilation (breast amputation, colostomy) is a source of mental distress and may inter-fere quite considerably with relationships between man and wife. By contrast, surgery which does not leave any obvious cosmetic deformity or defect appears not to have the same effect.

It appears that most mental distress amongst cancer patients is short-term and does not amount to formal psychiatric illness. Gener-ally, it takes the form of temporary feelings of depression, anxiety, and/or increased complaints of physical symptoms.

Psychiatric studies show that the amount of psychiatric illness in cancer is probably only slightly higher than in other chronic disorders that lead to hospitalization. About two thirds of the patients who suffer emotional distress have 'reactive depression/anxiety' caused by the illness and its effects upon them and their families. Very few patients (less than 10–15%) have major psychiatric illnesses. There-fore, the need for psychotropic drugs is not high. In the majority of patients, general measures of support with an explanation of the nature of the illness and its treatment, together with physical symptom relief, are all that is needed to bring about an improvement. Special attention should be paid to pain relief because the chances of mental distress developing are increased in the presence of chronic pain. This is particularly true if the patient believes that the pain is an indication of progressive disease which, of course, is not always the case.

PAIN AND EMOTIONAL CHANGE IN THE FOUR STAGES OF CANCER ILLNESS

There are four distinct phases, each with characteristic physical and emotional elements. The stages are:

(1)   Premedical contact

(2)   Medical investigation and diagnosis

(3)   Treatment

(4)   Post-treatment outcome.

Premedical contact

It is likely that most cancer sufferers are unaware of the nature of their illness prior to seeking medical attention unless a tumour mass is evident. Therefore, the reaction will be that of a previously healthy person who becomes afflicted by physical symptoms which may be unpleasant, debilitating and frightening.

   Amongst those who have some knowledge of illness and its possible causes the idea of cancer may develop despite the fact that there is little or no evidence for it. In many cases the initial reaction to a change from health to illness is one of anxiety with self-concern and worry about various bodily functions. Medical help may not be sought; many people turn to medicines which may be bought from pharmacies, or to those who prescribe traditional remedies that are not used by doctors. For a time anxiety may be reduced but the progression of symptoms will lead to increased anxiety and, at this point, medical help may be sought. In some cases, paradoxically, an established fear of cancer may delay consultation either because of overwhelming anxiety about the possible diagnosis, the investigation of the disorder and its treatment, or by the process of 'denial' in which the patient behaves as though the illness did not exist. In fact, he or she appears quite unconcerned by its presence; for example, a woman may say that an ulcerating tumour of the breast has been present for only a week or two, which is clearly not true. At this stage of illness the pain is likely to be mild to moderate, but unless it is adequately controlled its presence will increase emotional distress, chiefly by provoking anxiety, which in itself has the effect of further increasing pain.

Medical investigation and diagnosis

The emotions of both hope and fear are generated by medical examination.

To many patients the process of diagnosis is an unfamiliar and alarming experience which adds to their existing worries about health. Therefore, it is often with mixed emotions that they appear for discussion about diagnosis and treatment and the response of the doctor and his associates to the patient at this point is crucial.

Most patients and their relatives expect a clear but simple explanation of the disorder giving rise to the symptoms and an equally clear and reassuring statement about treatment required, its nature and effects, together with a general indication of the immediate outcome. The explanation should be clear and simple. If it is too complicated it will not be understood even by many intelligent patients, because of the anxiety surrounding the interview. With specific regard to pain it should be possible to describe the cause (for example pressure on nerves or obstruction to an abdominal organ) and to provide a good indication about the possibility of relief. The question of whether patients should be told that they have cancer is an issue of concern and debate in many countries. We consider that while the close relatives should be told the full truth, the patient should be told only as much as he wants to know.

Treatment

Treatments for cancer include surgery, radiotherapy, cytotoxic agents, hormones, and other drugs for symptomatic relief. All have powerful effects upon the body and in some cases the toxic effects are highly unpleasant and last for many weeks, even beyond the active phase of treatment. Permanent cosmetic changes may be produced by surgery and longlasting changes in appearance occur as the result of cytotoxic drugs and hormone therapy. Therefore it is often difficult to establish whether a disturbance of emotion in a patient is due to the effects of physical symptoms, to the effect of treatment, an emotional reaction to both, or an independent mental disorder. As stated previously, tiredness, lassitude, poor sleep, anorexia, and depression of mood are common, but are not necessarily indications of psychiatric illness.

A small proportion of patients will develop specific symptoms of a psychiatric nature. For example, true depressive illness presents with a deep and persistent lowering of mood, abnormal feelings of guilt and suicidal thoughts, none of which is corrected by the relief of physical symptoms, or simple psychological support. In such patients, especially men, there is a definite risk of suicide and this is increased if pain is a major symptom. Specific antidepressant therapy will be needed and the doctor should prescribe drugs which produce the lowest level of side-effects in order to avoid further distressing physical symptoms (see p. 86).

There is a relationship between the treatment of malignant disease and psychiatric symptoms of depression and anxiety. Thus in women who undergo mastectomy alone for treatment, up to 50% will develop depression, anxiety and sexual difficulties. This percentage is increased to 80% if cytotoxic drugs are also used. Moreover, these problems persist for a long time after treatment and are associated with emotional distress in the patient's husband. However, the level of morbidity may be reduced dramatically if simple counselling is carried out by nurses who have had a basic training designed to help them discuss patient's symptoms and their control, and family and marital problems. The effects of counselling have also been observed in other conditions, for example amongst patients who have colostomies after surgery for malignant disease of the bowel.

Other psychiatric disorders, apart from depression and anxiety, may appear at this stage and they include the organic brain syndrome, or organic confusion state (which may be the result of the disease, or the toxic effects of drugs used in its treatment) and sexual disorders (which arise as part of the general debility or as a consequence of the effects of treatment, or for psychological reasons associated with physical mutilation caused by the disease and/or treatment).

It is clear that the management of cancer patients in pain during the stage of active treatment is unlikely to be completely successful unless both symptom control and psychological support are given full attention (see Continuing Care, p. 64).

Post-treatment outcome

For some patients treatment of the primary malignancy will have a definite end-point as, for example, following surgery for neoplasm of the bowel. In other cases maintenance treatment is needed for months, years, or the remainder of the patient's life. Alternatively, following acute treatment, there may be steady progression of the disease or an interval of freedom before the development of fresh symptoms indicating metastatic spread of the primary tumour. With the progression of malignant disease, whether continuous with the primary illness or following a symptom-free period, the likelihood of pain increases.

Experts in pain control, using the best methods available (which means both physical and psychological techniques) are able to reduce the number of individuals suffering very severe pain to a very small proportion of those in the terminal stages of illness, demonstrating that good control can be achieved with appropriate facilities. Such facilities are not always available which means that the physical and emotional burdens of the sufferers will be high. Pain is not the only symptom to cause extreme distress. Others in this category include vomiting, dyspnoea, and itching in particular. To make sense of the many possible emotional problems that may occur it is worth considering them in terms of the nature of the outcome of treatment.

Total relief of physical symptoms

In the case of the removal of an obstructive tumour of the bowel where anxiety accompanied the initial acute painful symptoms, relief is followed by rapid, physical and emotional recovery. Later the appearance of new symptoms, including pain, anorexia, weight loss, jaundice, or vomiting, is accompanied by fresh feelings of anxiety and fear as the patient moves into what may be the terminal phase of the illness.

Freedom from physical symptoms with residual cosmetic defects

In Western countries facial or bodily disfigurement by surgery often provokes feelings of depression and despair and may lead to partial or even complete withdrawal from social contact other than with family members and close friends. It is not unknown for a fully developed depressive illness to occur in such circumstances and sexual impotence in men and loss of libido in both sexes is quite common. The extent to which these phenomena are a problem for postsurgical patients in other countries varies considerably but, if present, it produces not only personal distress for the patient, but also for the family and, in particular, the husband or wife. Clearly an awareness of this possibility is essential when dealing with postsurgical emotional disorders.

Residual or increasing physical symptoms including pain

Advanced malignant disease is physically debilitating and the prevailing feelings of many patients are those of depression and fear. The appearance of fresh symptoms, especially if difficult to control medically, usually produces an upsurge in emotion with anxiety predominating as many patients regard such events as evidence of disease progression, although this may not be the case. Therefore, it is important that doctors and nurses talk to patients and relatives about symptom control, reassuring them that they do not indicate progression of disease (if this is true) and giving a realistic view of the chances of controlling the symptom, including a brief description of the treatment needed.

THE MANAGEMENT OF EMOTIONAL DISORDERS

Communication with patients and relatives

Doctors vary in their ability to appreciate and understand the emotional problems of their patients and they have differing views about the extent to which they should discuss illness with patients. Patients also differ in their opinions about the extent to which they should discuss their problems with a doctor.

In view of these problems it is worth mentioning those qualities that have been identified as contributing positively towards doctor/patient relationships. They are, first, that the doctor is 'psychologically oriented'. In other words he is interested in the emotions of others, recognizes changes in them and has the ability to appreciate their depth and meaning. Next, the doctor encourages the patient to talk about his emotions and has the ability to listen rather than conduct the interview through a series of direct questions. Third, if the doctor can understand the patient's psychological problems he is more likely to solve social and family emotional problems by discussion rather than by the use of drugs.

These qualities appear to be part of a doctor's personality but they may be acquired to a considerable extent by conscious effort and training. In the management of cancer patients they are a very necessary part of the approach to care and should form the background to the attitude taken by the management team, irrespective of its size. It is found that within such teams the possession of these qualities is not equal and the person dealing chiefly with emotional and social problems may not, therefore, be the doctor although the doctor is always the team leader. Dealing with patients' disturbed emotions has effects upon those caring for them. Awareness of this fact and discussion between members of the treatment team of the problems they have encountered is common practice in specialized centres and is known to reduce tension amongst the carers themselves. Events likely to produce difficulties for the carers include the presence of an emotionally disturbed patient, difficulties with relatives, patient's death, and differences of opinion between team members about management practices. It should be pointed out that often the patient's relatives become emotionally disturbed, and require clear communication and sensitive handling.

The use of drugs for management of emotional disturbance

Psychotropic drugs are used in only a small proportion of cases to deal specifically with emotional disturbances. Anxiolytics are used more frequently than antidepressants and chiefly for the control of minor states of tension or anxiety. Neither group of drugs appears to be used to any extent in the direct control of pain, although the neuroleptics or major tranquillizers are used to a limited extent as adjuvants to narcotic analgesics (see Chapter 7).

Psychological techniques for pain relief

Psychological methods that have been used in pain relief are:

(1)   Psychotherapy for individuals or groups of individuals

(2)　Hypnotherapy

(3)　Modification of pain behaviour by operant conditioning

(4)　Biofeedback and relaxation.

Psychotherapy

Of the techniques available those offering most value in the treatment of patients with cancer pain in terms of their applicability under all circumstances are psychotherapy and hypnotherapy. The term psychotherapy covers methods ranging from simple and direct counselling to psychoanalysis. Clearly it is only the simpler forms of therapy that are relevant to this text and, in fact, there is little good evidence that the more elaborate techniques are more effective.

Counselling, alternatively known as supportive psychotherapy, is based on a process involving listening carefully to a patient's conversation and showing understanding and concern, if appropriate, as the latter puts forward problems, conflicts and anxieties. Reassurance and advice are given and the doctor uses his own experience in life to help the patient gain a clearer understanding of the situation.

This form of therapy is frequently used, consciously or otherwise, by many doctors and is of considerable value in dealing with patients with acute or chronic illnesses.

Following the principles of supportive psychotherapy at an early stage the doctor should give the patient a simple factual explanation of the illness, the treatment he intends to carry out and his expectations about the outcome, being honest about any unpleasant effects the treatment may bring, for example the fact that pain may occur but that it will be minimized if not abolished by appropriate drugs. During the course of illnesses due to cancer, acute exacerbations of symptoms occur producing anxiety and a sense of disorganization for the patient, who requires the doctor's support in order to establish a sense of orderliness by labelling the cause of the disturbance which the doctor should treat promptly. This provides a new self-image for the patient and the relief gained from treatment consolidates the relationship between doctor and patient. Although it is common for supportive psychotherapy to be carried out with individual patients there are occasions when group psychotherapy has advantages. For example, such a technique reduces a patient's sense of being alone, of being alienated, and of being different because he is in the presence of others with similar physical, emotional and social difficulties. Patients are often more willing to accept interpretation of their difficulties and advice about their management from fellow patients than from the doctor. Their fears about the nature of the disease, lifelong incapacity, the possibility of death, their ability to cope with stress, and other problems, are subjects that often arise spontaneously in discussion and, as they do so, the group gives support or criticism to one or more of its members. This technique may add considerable support to the doctor's own efforts carried on outside the group by helping the patient to establish sensible goals in terms of work, leisure and personal relationships. Also they are encouraged to develop realistic attitudes towards their future and what they will eventually be able to achieve, even though this may be a much lower level of activity than before the illness began.

Hypnotherapy

Hypnotherapy is a state of mind in which the subject shows increased susceptibility to suggestions made by the hypnotist. It appears that a hypnotic trance is most easily induced in subjects who have a highly developed ability to produce mental images suggested to them by the therapist and that hypnotizability is an aspect of each person's personality which does not change appreciably from childhood to old age. The hypnotist can vary the response of the subject by inducing a state which varies from a mild degree of hypersuggestibility to one in which physical changes, such as anaesthesia, can be induced. There is no doubt that a number of patients when hypnotized can endure physical experiences which would normally be painful and of course it can be used as an adjunct to mild or moderate analgesics, which is particularly useful in those countries where potent narcotics are not available. It is often said that the number of individuals in any given society who are susceptible to hypnosis is quite small, but in fact the number who can benefit from the techniques of hypnotherapy is quite large because the state of calm, relaxation, and distraction from noxious stimuli is of benefit to many patients who have pain which is intensified by fear, unpleasant memories or thoughts. However, there are very few practical hypnotherapists available.

It is not the purpose of this book to describe the techniques of hypnotherapy in detail and the reader should refer to a more comprehensive text for this purpose and seek training if needed (see Recommended reading).

The techniques of behaviour modification and biofeedback have been used only to a limited extent in patients with cancer pain and their effectiveness has not yet been proven.

The use of acupuncture, other than in areas of the world where it has a long established place in the management of painful disorders, is not advised because the reliability of the technique is low.

Recommended reading

1. Shone, R. (ed.) (1982). *Autohypnosis.* (Wellingborough, UK: Thorsons Ltd.).
2. Swerdlow, M. (ed.) (1986) *Therapy of Pain*, 2nd Edn. (Lancaster: MTP Press)

PART TWO
Assessment

4

Assessment of Pain in Patients with Cancer

K. M. Foley

When we are evaluating a patient with pain and cancer, a detailed psychological and social history, combined with a complete medical and neurological examination provide the most essential information. By defining the type of pain, its site, its exacerbating and relieving factors and its associated clinical signs the physician can make a provisional diagnosis of the cause or causes of the pain. He can then order the necessary investigations to confirm the clinical diagnosis and employ the appropriate treatment to manage the pain.

In the dying patient the physician may choose to decide the cause clinically and treat it empirically. In the newly diagnosed, untreated cancer patient, however, this empirical approach must be discouraged because assessment and treatment of the cause of the pain are the best approach.

To fully assess the cancer patient with pain, the physician needs to familiarize himself with:

(1) The types of pain

(2) The types of patients with pain

(3) The common pain syndromes in cancer patients (see Chapter 5)

(4) The psychological and social factors which are involved in the pain complaint.

TYPES OF PAIN

Cancer patients may have both acute and chronic pain. Increased understanding of pain mechanisms has shown that the central modulation for these two types of pain may be different. In clinical practice the distinction between acute and chronic pain is particularly important because management of patients with these two types of pain and their response to treatment are often quite different.

Acute pain is relatively easy to recognize and is often more amenable to relief particularly by treatment of the cause. (The point at which acute pain becomes chronic is not known but pain lasting for longer than 1–6 months is usually considered to be chronic pain.)

With patients in *chronic pain* the persistent pain has usually failed to respond to the treatment of the cause. In these patients, the pain has led to significant changes in personality, lifestyle and functional ability. These patients need a thorough assessment of the pain complaint: the physician should respect the complaint and by a careful history and examination define its physical and psychological dimensions. It is very important to define both the sensory component of the pain and the emotional impact. In defining the sensory component of the pain, the doctor must note both the severity and the quality.

With regard to the *severity*, the doctor should ask the patient to define the pain as mild, moderate or severe.

The *quality* of pain often varies and may be described as dull or sharp, localized or diffuse, aching, burning or cramping, continuous or intermittent. It is important to get the patient to describe the quality of the pain because this will give valuable information about the cause. For example *incident pain* is characterized by no pain at rest with an acute exacerbation of pain on change of position and suggests the presence of a pathological fracture. Pain associated with nerve injury is often described as burning and dysaesthetic with sensations of coldness or heat. The various types of pain are described on pages 45–54.

TYPES OF PATIENTS WITH PAIN

It is useful to recognize that there are different classes of patients with pain as well as common pain syndromes. Patients can be classified into three groups.

Group I – patients with acute pain

If the pain is associated with the diagnosis of cancer it has a special significance as the harbinger of that illness. Recurrent pain during the course of cancer or following initial therapy also has the implications of recurrence of the disease. However, effective treatment of the cause of the pain can result in dramatic pain relief in a majority of patients.

On the other hand, if the acute pain is associated with cancer therapy, the cause of pain is readily identifiable and is self-limited. Pain treatment should be directed at the cause of the pain and analgesic drug therapy is used to manage the transient symptoms. These patients will often endure a significant amount of pain if they are assured of a successful outcome. This emphasizes how the significance of pain can markedly alter the patient's ability to tolerate it.

Group II – patients with chronic pain

Pain associated with progression of the disease

The pain escalates in intensity with tumour infiltration of adjacent bone, nerve or soft tissue. Combinations of antitumour therapy, analgesic drug therapy, anaesthetic blocks, neurosurgical approaches (and alternative methods of pain control) are all relevant and have varying rates of success. Psychological factors play a significant role in this group of patients. Palliative therapy can help but it may be of little value and may be physically debilitating.

Hopelessness and fear of death may further add to and exaggerate the pain complaint. Management must be directed at the treatment of pain, recognizing that treatment of the cause of the pain has failed. This is true for the majority of patients with advanced cancer pain.

Pain associated with cancer therapy

The pain is often secondary to soft tissue, nerve or bony injury caused most commonly by surgery or chemotherapy and is not related to tumour infiltration. For these patients treatment should also be directed at the symptoms, not the cause. It is important to identify this group of patients because recognition that the pain is not caused by tumour growth markedly alters the patient's therapy, prognosis and psychological state. Each of the primary methods of cancer therapy is associated with a specific chronic pain syndrome having a characteristic pain pattern and clinical presentation (see Chapter 5).

Group III – dying patients with pain

In this group the physician's goal should be to maintain the comfort of the patient (see Chapter 12). The issues of hopelessness, death and dying become prominent and the suffering component must be attended to. Inadequate control of pain further exacerbates the suffering component and demoralizes both the family and care givers who feel that they have failed in treating the patient's pain at a time when adequate treatment may have mattered most. Analgesic drug therapy should be rapidly escalated and psychological symptoms should be adequately improved.

Before considering the common pain syndromes which occur in cancer patients, certain general principles are summarized below. Lack of attention to these principles is the main reason for wrong diagnosis.

General principles of pain assessment

(1) Take a careful history of the pain complaint, which must be believed.

(2) Assess the psychosocial status of the patient.

(3) Perform a careful medical and neurological examination.

(4) Order and personally review the appropriate diagnostic procedures.

(5) Evaluate the extent of the patient's disease.

(6) Treat the pain to facilitate any diagnostic procedure.

(7) Consider all methods of pain control during the initial evaluation.

(8) Reassess the pain and the response to treatment during the course of therapy.

(1) Take a careful history of the pain complaint

The establishment of a trusting relationship with the physician is critical to the management of the patient with cancer. You must take the patient's complaint seriously and assess its reality and severity. The complaint of pain is a symptom, not a diagnosis. It is not simply a question of the amount of physical injury sustained by the patient but a complex state determined by multiple factors including age, sex, cultural and environmental influences, medical history and psychological factors.

There are certain characteristic descriptions of pain that can help to decide on the cause. A diagnosis is often made on the following criteria of pain: the onset, duration, characteristics, referral patterns, exacerbating and relieving factors, and associated signs and symptoms. For example, in a patient complaining of severe elbow pain exacerbated by coughing, the finding of a Horner's syndrome indicates paraspinal involvement of the tumour at the T1 vertebral level. Another common example is the cancer patient with severe back pain who complains of difficulty in urinating. These symptoms suggest the diagnosis of epidural spinal cord compression. Multiple pain complaints are common in patients with advanced disease and these need to be classified according to their degree of importance. It is also necessary to verify the history from a family member who may provide information that the patient is unable or unwilling to provide. For example, if the patient minimizes his symptoms, family members may give a more objective assessment of the patient's disability. Similarly, if the patient gives an inadequate history, a family member may be able to provide essential information that may alter the diagnostic approach. In short, all attempts should be made to obtain an adequate detailed history.

(2)   Assess the psychosocial status of the patient

The history should include the patient's previous record of anxiety or depression, suicidal ideation and degree of physical disability.

Psychological factors play a significant part in accounting for differences in pain experience in patients with cancer (see Chapter 3). A clear understanding of the functional level of the patient and his social environment is also necessary. Does the patient live alone or is there a responsible friend or relative who cares for him? Can he perform the normal activities of his daily living or does he require assistance? Is he still working? Does he comply with medical advice? It is important to recognize these factors to ensure that pain treatment is successful but does not interfere with the patient's functional activity.

(3) Perform a careful medical and neurological examination

The medical and neurological examinations help to provide the necessary data to substantiate the clinical history. Knowledge of the referral patterns of pain and the common pain syndromes can direct the examination. Areas of sensory loss or hyperaesthesia should be mapped out. Changes in reflexes, muscular weakness and/or atrophy can help to define the segmental level of nerve dysfunction. For example, in a patient with tumour infiltration of the chest wall, the dermatomal pattern of sensory loss can be used to envisage the extent of local tumour infiltration. In a patient with nerve injury pain from tumour infiltration, hyperpathia in an area of sensory loss is common and is detected clinically by increased sensibility to pinprick and light touch.

However, it is not uncommon for patients with significant cancer pain to have a normal physical or neurological examination. This is most common in patients with early tumour infiltration of the brachial, lumbar or sacral plexus or in patients with retroperitoneal tumour. Often they will complain of pain for several weeks or months before any evidence of objective physical, or neurological abnormality can be detected. In such instances, the history and the physician's judgement of the clinical diagnosis will decide which diagnostic investigations are needed.

(4) Order and personally review the appropriate diagnostic procedures

Since the diagnosis of metastatic disease may be difficult the physician ordering such studies should recognize the limitations of the available diagnostic procedures. It is important to ensure that visualization of the area under study is as adequate as possible.

Plain X-rays are a useful screening procedure, but they may not show any abnormalities despite the presence of bony metastases. There must be a 40–60% change in bone density to detect a tumour by X-ray and pain can occur in the absence of such extensive destruction. Often 3–4 months elapse before changes appear on the plain film. The bone scan, if available, provides a more sensitive method of demonstrating abnormalities.

More specialized techniques such as computerized transaxial tomography, if available, allow for detailed visualization of soft tissue and bone. This method is the procedure of choice in evaluating patients with brachial, lumbar or sacral plexus pain complaints. Cisternal and lumbar myelography and cerebrospinal fluid evaluation are the other diagnostic procedures which can further help diagnosis.

(5)   Evaluate the extent of the patient's disease

Evaluation of the extent of metastatic disease may help to decide whether the pain is due to recurrent disease. For example, the post-mastectomy pain syndrome which occurs secondary to interruption of the intercostobrachial nerve is never caused by recurrent disease. In contrast, in the patient with carcinoma of the lung, following initial resolution of the postoperative pain, the appearance of post-thoracotomy pain is likely to be due to recurrent disease.

(6)   Treat the pain to facilitate the diagnostic investigation

Analgesic drug therapy should be used for initial pain relief. The patient should not be inadequately evaluated because he is in significant pain. If the pain is controlled while the source is being investigated he will more easily be able to participate in the necessary diagnostic procedures.

(7)   Consider all methods of pain control during the initial evaluation

Analgesic drug therapy is the mainstay of pain management, but the use of other methods of pain control should also be considered early on. For example, a cordotomy can provide the patient with significant relief from pain in one leg due to tumour infiltration of the lumbosacral plexus.

The use of local anaesthetic or neurolytic blocks similarly can provide adequate pain relief in the patient with localized pain.

Physical therapy, including adequate bracing to facilitate ambulation and reduce incident pain, can play an important role.

(8)   Reassess the pain and the response to treatment during the course of therapy

Continual reassessment of the patient's response to treatment is the best way to check that the initial diagnosis was correct.

If the response to therapy is less than expected, or if exacerbation of the pain occurs, you should reassess the treatment or search for a new cause of the pain, for example, the patient with vertebral body bony disease who develops increasing local pain from an epidural cord compression.

Recommended reading

1. Bonica, J. J. and Ventafridda, V. (eds.) (1979). *Advances in Pain Research and Therapy*, Vol. 2 (New York: Raven Press)
2. Twycross, R. G. and Lack, S. A. (1983). *Symptom Control in Far Advanced Cancer: Pain Relief*. (London: Pitman)
3. Foley, K. M. (1985). The treatment of cancer pain. *N. Engl. J. Med.*, **313**, 84–95
4. Foley, K. M. and Sundaresan, N. (1985). The management of cancer pain. In Devita, V. T., Hellman, S. and Rosenberg, S. A. (eds.) *Cancer Principles and Practice in Oncology*, pp. 1940–1965. (New York: Lippincott)

5

Pain Syndromes in Patients with Cancer

K. M. Foley

Establishing an accurate diagnosis is the key to providing the right treatment.

PAIN ASSOCIATED WITH DIRECT TUMOUR INVOLVEMENT

Tumour infiltration of bone

Pain from invasion of bone by either primary or metastatic tumour is the most common cause of pain in patients with cancer. The pain may be the presenting complaint, e.g. in patients with multiple myeloma, or it may represent the first sign of metastatic disease, e.g. patients with carcinoma of the breast. The patient may have his pain at the site of the lesion, e.g. rib pain, or the pain may be referred to a distant area of the body, e.g. knee pain associated with metastatic hip disease. The characteristics of the pain vary with the site involved, but in general the pain is constant and usually grows progressively more severe.

Metastases to the base of the skull

These syndromes all share two common features. Pain is the earliest complaint, often preceding neurological signs and symptoms by several weeks to months, and diagnosis with plain X-rays is often difficult.

Syndromes

Jugular foramen syndrome – Occipital pain, often referred to the vertex of the head and ipsilateral shoulder and arm, is an early presenting symptom. The pain is often exacerbated by head movement and associated with local tenderness over the occipital condyle. The patient's signs and symptoms vary with the cranial nerve involved, but can include hoarseness, dysarthria, dysphagia, neck and shoulder weakness, and ptosis. The neurological examination can help to localize the lesion by determining the function of the IXth, Xth, and XIIth cranial nerves, since involvement of all four of these nerves suggests jugular foramen and hypoglossal-canal involvement with secondary nerve dysfunction. The presence of a Horner's syndrome suggests sympathetic involvement extracranially but in close proximity to the jugular foramen.

Clivus metastases – These commonly cause pain characterized by a vertex headache which is exacerbated by neck flexion. Lower cranial nerve dysfunction (VI–XIIth) usually begins unilaterally, but often progresses to bilateral lower cranial nerve dysfunction.

Sphenoid-sinus metastases – These give rise to severe bifrontal headache radiating to both temples, with intermittent retro-orbital pain. The patient often complains of nasal stuffiness or a sense of fullness in the head, with concomitant diplopia. The neurological sign of unilateral or bilateral VIth nerve palsy helps further to suggest the diagnosis.

Metastases to vertebral bodies

These syndromes share the common feature of pain as an early symptom which, if not accurately diagnosed, may lead to irreversible neurological deficits, e.g. paraplegia.

Cervical vertebrae

C1–C2 subluxation – Metastatic disease involving the odontoid process of the axis (C1 vertebral body) can result in a pathological fracture with secondary subluxation resulting in spinal cord or brainstem compression. The early symptoms include severe neck pain radiating over the posterior aspect of the skull to the vertex, exacerbated by movement, particularly flexion of the neck. Neurological signs include progressive sensory and motor signs beginning in the upper extremities with associated autonomic dysfunction. Neck manipulation in these patients is dangerous. Tomography is generally necessary to confirm the diagnosis.

C7–T1 metastases – Pain due to metastatic disease to the C7–T1 vertebral bodies is usually localized to the adjacent paraspinal area and characterized by a constant, dull, aching pain radiating to both shoulders. There may be tenderness to percussion over the spinous process at this level. With nerve root compression, radicular pain in the C7–C8–T1 distribution occurs most commonly unilaterally in the posterior arm, elbow, and ulnar aspect of the hand. The neurological symptoms include paraesthesiae and numbness in the 4th and 5th fingers, with progressive hand weakness and triceps weakness. The presence of a Horner's syndrome suggests paravertebral sympathetic involvement. Metastatic bone disease at this level results from either haematogenous spread to bone or, more commonly, from tumour originating in the brachial plexus or paravertebral space and spreading along the nerves to the contiguous vertebral body and epidural space.

Lumbar

L1 metastases – Dull, aching mid-back pain exacerbated by lying or sitting and relieved by standing is the usual presenting complaint. Radicular pain in a girdle-like manner anteriorly or to both paraspinal lumbosacral areas may also be present. Occasionally patients will have only pain referred to the sacroiliac joint and/or the superior iliac crest.

Sacral metastases – Aching pain, beginning insidiously, in the low back or coccygeal region, and exacerbated by lying or sitting and relieved by walking is the common clinical complaint. Increasing pain, with the neurological signs and symptoms of perianal sensory loss, bowel and bladder dysfunction, and impotence help to localize the site of disease.

Degenerative disc disease rarely occurs at the C7–T1 or L1 areas; this fact should suggest a need for further investigation of pain complaints involving these areas. Osteoporosis can often mimic the signs and symptoms of metastatic bone disease.

Epidural spinal cord compression – This is associated with vertebral body metastases in 85% of patients, and a careful neurological history and examination can help to establish evidence of spinal cord dysfunction. If there are signs of neurological dysfunction, myelography should be performed to delineate the extent of epidural disease.

SIGNS AND SYMPTOMS OF TUMOUR INFILTRATION OF NERVES

Tumour infiltration of peripheral nerve

Constant, burning pain with hyperaesthesia and dysaesthesia in the area of sensory loss is the usual clinical presentation. Tumour compression of proximal peripheral nerves occurs most commonly in association with paravertebral or retroperitoneal tumour. The pain is radicular and unilateral, and a careful sensory examination can often delineate the site of nerve compression. Metastatic tumour in rib often produces intercostal nerve involvement; pain is the earliest symptom, with progressive sensory loss distal to the site of nerve compression.

Tumour infiltration of brachial plexus

This syndrome, often referred to as the superior pulmonary sulcus or Pancoast syndrome, results from tumour infiltration of the lower brachial plexus. It is characterized by pain radiating to the ipsilateral shoulder, posterior aspect of the arm and elbow, in a C8–T1 distribution. The neurological symptoms of pain and paraesthesiae in the fourth and fifth fingers may precede objective clinical signs by several weeks to months. These paraesthesiae progress to numbness and weakness in a C7–C8–T1 distribution. The supraclavicular and axillary regions may be normal. The presence of a Horner's syndrome suggests involvement of the sympathetic chain in the paravertebral space.

Lumbar plexus tumour infiltration

This occurs most commonly in patients with genitourinary, gynae-cological and colonic cancers from local tumour extension into adjacent lymph nodes and bone. The pain varies with the site of plexus involvement and is generally of two types: radicular pain in the anterior thigh and groin (L1–2–3 distribution), or down the posterior aspect of the leg to the heel (L5–S1 distribution). Referred pain without local pain may also occur and presents a more difficult diagnostic problem. Pain in the anterior thigh, lateral aspect of the calf or heel associated with palpable local tenderness represents referred pain from lumbar plexus tumour infiltration. The neurological symptoms include paraesthesiae followed by numbness and dysaesthesiae with progressive motor and sensory loss in a plexus distribution. The presence of asymmetric or absent reflexes on neurological examination often suggests root involvement. The absence of palpable tumour in the pelvis or groin does not preclude the diagnosis.

Sacral plexus tumour infiltration

This occurs most commonly in patients with colonic, genitourinary or gynaecological cancers. Dull, aching midline pain with sensory loss beginning in the perineal area is the usual clinical presentation. The sensory findings are initially unilateral, but progress to bilateral sacral sensory loss and autonomic dysfunction including impotence and bowel and bladder dysfunction.

Meningeal carcinomatosis

In this syndrome there is tumour infiltration of the cerebrospinal leptomeninges with or without concomitant invasion of the parenchyma of the nervous system. Pain occurs in 40% of patients and is generally of two types: (a) headache with or without neck stiffness characterized by a constant pain: and (b) back pain most commonly localized to the low back and buttock regions. Pain results from traction on tumour-infiltrated nerves and meninges.

Epidural spinal cord compression

Severe neck and back pain is the hallmark of this condition. Pain is the initial symptom in 96% of patients, and in 10% is the only symptom. The pain results from local bone or root compression and is radicular. It is generally unilateral in patients with cervical or lumbosacral compression but bilateral if the thoracic cord is compressed. The neurological symptoms vary with the site of epidural disease and commonly include motor weakness progressing to paraplegia, sensory loss, and loss of bowel and bladder function.

Most patients with epidural cord compression also have vertebral body tumour.

PAIN SYNDROMES ASSOCIATED WITH CANCER THERAPY

Clinical pain syndromes occur in the course of, or subsequent to, treatment of cancer patients with surgery, chemotherapy or radiation therapy.

Postsurgery pain

Post-thoracotomy pain

Pain in the distribution of an intercostal nerve occurs in a small percentage of patients following thoracotomy. Pain becomes evident 1–2 months after the surgical procedure and is characterized by a constant pain in the area of sensory loss with occasional intermittent lancinating pains. Dysaesthesia in the scar area, with hyperaesthesia in the surrounding zone, are often prominent symptoms. Movement exacerbates the pain, and the patient may develop a concomitant frozen shoulder characterized by limitation of movement at the shoulder joint and disuse atrophy of the arm. Early recognition of this syndrome and its sequelae can often prevent the development of further limitation of shoulder movement.

Postmastectomy pain

Pain in the posterior arm, axilla, and anterior chest wall in patients following radical mastectomy occurs from interruption of the inter-costobrachial nerve, a cutaneous branch of T1 nerve. The onset of pain is usually 1–2 months after the surgical procedure and is more common in patients whose postoperative course is complicated by either excessive local swelling or infection. The pain is characterized as a tight, constricting, burning pain in the posterior arm and axilla which radiates across the anterior chest wall. There is usually no associated lymphoedema of the arm. The pain is exacerbated by arm movement, and patients often keep the arm in a flexed position close to the chest wall. As with post-thoracotomy pain, a frozen shoulder may develop, producing a second problem of increased pain and limitation of movement at the shoulder joint.

Postradical neck dissection pain

Pain following radical neck dissection occurs from surgical injury or interruption of the cervical nerves. The pain is characterized by a constant burning sensation in the area of sensory loss. Dysaesthesiae and intermittent shock-like pain may also be present.

Phantom-limb pain

Pain following surgical amputation of a limb is generally either stump pain or phantom-limb pain. These painful clinical conditions are different from *phantom-limb sensation*, which occurs in all patients following limb amputation. The phantom-limb pain is usually characterized by a burning, cramping pain in the phantom limb, often identical in nature and location to the preoperative pain.

Postchemotherapy pain

A series of pain problems can occur in cancer patients receiving chemotherapy. The major features of each of these entities is briefly described below.

Peripheral neuropathy – Painful dysaesthesiae following treatment with the Vinca alkaloid drugs occur as part of a symmetrical polyneuropathy. Both vincristine and vinblastine are neurotoxic drugs in the doses required to achieve an antineoplastic effect. The dysaesthesiae are commonly localized to the hands and feet, and are characterized by burning pain exacerbated by superficial stimuli.

Steroid pseudo-rheumatism – This occurs from both rapid and slow withdrawal of steroid medications in patients taking these drugs for either short or long periods of time. The syndrome consists of prominent diffuse myalgias and arthralgias, with muscle and joint tenderness on palpation but without objective inflammatory signs. A sense of generalized malaise and fatigue is a common feature. These signs and symptoms revert if steroid medication is restarted.

Aseptic necrosis of bone – Both aseptic necrosis of the humoral and, much more commonly, the femoral head are complications of cancer therapy, specifically chronic steroid therapy. Pain in the shoulder or knee and leg are the common presenting complaints, with X-ray changes occurring several weeks to months after the onset of pain. There is limitation of joint movements, with progressive inability to use the arm or hip. Aseptic bone necrosis occurs most commonly in patients with Hodgkin's disease, although it can occur in any patient on chronic steroid therapy.

Postradiation therapy pain

Radiation fibrosis of the brachial plexus

Pain in the distribution of the brachial plexus following radiation therapy occurs from fibrosis of the surrounding connective tissue and secondary injury to nerve. It may appear as early as 6 months or as late as 20 years after radiation treatment. It presents a difficult diagnostic problem in that it must be differentiated from recurrent tumour. The clinical symptoms include complaints of numbness or paraesthesiae in the hand, usually in a C5–6 distribution. Pain occurs later, often as diffuse arm pain. Lymphoedema in the arm and radiation skin changes and induration of the supraclavicular and axillary areas are often present. The neurological signs include sensory changes in a C5–6–7 distribution, with motor weakness most prominent in the deltoid and biceps muscles. These signs progress to the development of a painful, useless, swollen extremity. In contrast, with tumour infiltration of the brachial plexus pain is the earliest symptom, with sensory changes in a C8–T1 distribution and motor weakness beginning distally rather than proximally. The associated signs with radiation injury include evidence on X-ray of radiation injury to the lung, rib, or humerus. These findings may help to confirm a history of radiation injury in the absence of appropriate radiation data.

Radiation fibrosis of the lumbar plexus

Pain in the leg from radiation fibrosis of the lumbar plexus presents a similar diagnostic problem of radiation injury versus recurrent tumour. Pain occurring late in the course of progressive motor and sensory changes in the leg is more common with radiation fibrosis but is not the most reliable clinical symptom. A previous history of radiation treatment and local skin changes or lymphoedema of the leg with X-ray changes demonstrating radiation necrosis of bone may help to establish this diagnosis.

The diagnostic investigation to differentiate nerve fibrosis from nerve infiltration by tumour should include plain X-rays of the area to delineate radiation changes in bone or evidence of recurrent metastatic disease. In some cases, surgical exploration may be necessary, particularly in patients free of known metastatic disease, to determine further cancer management.

Radiation myelopathy

Pain is an early symptom in 15% of patients with this condition and may be localized to the area of spinal cord damage or referred, with dysaesthesiae below the level of injury. Clinically, the neurological signs and symptoms are those of a Brown–Sequard syndrome (ipsilateral motor paresis with contralateral sensory loss at a cervical or thoracic level) which progresses to a complete transverse myelopathy. The diagnostic investigation should include careful plain X-rays of the spine and myelography, both of which are usually normal. Occasionally, widening of the cord at the injured area may be noted.

Radiation-induced peripheral nerve tumours

A painful, enlarging mass in an area of previous irradiation can occur many years after radiation therapy. Patients usually present with pain and a progressive neurological deficit, with a palpable mass involving the brachial or lumbar plexus. Surgical exploration and biopsy is necessary to establish the diagnosis. The important differential diagnoses include radiation fibrosis and recurrent tumour.

PAIN UNRELATED TO CANCER OR CANCER THERAPY

Approximately 3% of the pain syndromes which occur in cancer patients have no relationship to the underlying cancer or cancer therapy. The commonest of these non-cancer pain syndromes are degenerative disc disease, thoracic and abdominal aneurysms and diffuse osteoporosis. This emphasizes the point that pain in a cancer patient does not necessarily imply recurrent or persistent disease. A careful diagnostic evaluation of the cancer patient is essential to define the specific pain syndrome before embarking on treatment.

Postherpetic neuralgia

This is a well-described condition characterized by pain which persists after the cutaneous eruption from herpes zoster infection has cleared. In patients with cancer, herpes zoster infection commonly occurs in the area of tumour pathology or in the part of previous radiation therapy. The true incidence of postherpetic neuralgia in patients with cancer is unknown, but it appears to be more common in patients who develop the infection after the age of 50. There are generally three types of pain: (a) a continuous, burning pain in the area of sensory loss, (b) painful dysaesthesiae, and (c) intermittent, lancinating pain.

Recommended reading

1. Bonica, J. J. and Ventafridda, V. (eds.) (1979). *Advances in Pain Research and Therapy*, Vol. 2 (New York: Raven Press).
2. Foley, K. M. (1985). The treatment of cancer pain. *N. Engl. J. Med.*, **313**, 84–95.
3. Foley, K. M. (1985). The control of pain in cancer. In Calabrisi, P., Schein, P. and Rosenberg, S. (eds.) *Medical Oncology: Basic Principles and Clinical Management of Cancer*, pp. 1385–1405 (New York: Macmillan).

PART THREE
Treatment

6

Therapeutic Strategy

V. Ventafridda

We have now determined, as far as possible, the nature and cause of the pain and we must decide how we can best relieve it.

The first step must be to treat the cause of the pain if this is possible. If there is no available treatment for the cause of the pain, the management of the pain itself becomes the physician's primary objective.

In choosing the method(s) of treatment, you must bear in mind the patient's degree of activity. If he complains of severe pain but has a full range of life activities make sure that the planned pain relieving method will interfere as little as possible with activity. On the other hand, if pain is interfering considerably with the quality of his life (eating, sleeping, performance status, social activity) the pain must be treated actively and radically.

The therapeutic strategy must be based on (1) immediate action to relieve pain; and then (2) continuous control for the remainder of the patient's life. The ideal goal of this strategy – complete freedom from pain – is rarely possible but pain can always be eased so that the patient can bear what was previously considered to be intolerable suffering.

In planning the therapeutic strategy we must pursue a series of objectives:

(1)   Increase the hours of sleep. Cancer pain may prevent the patient

from getting adequate sleep, which will lower his pain threshold and result in constant tiredness and demoralization.

(2)   Then relieve pain when resting in bed or chair.

(3)   Then relieve pain felt when standing and during activity.

While the first and the second aims are relatively easy to achieve, the third one requires a combined and sequential pattern of physical and psychosocial supports to be adequately effective. This sequence foresees the use of the least harmful, most simple and most effective available modalities for the relief of the patient's pain (Figure 6).

INITIAL APPROACH

The pain should first be alleviated as far as possible with analgesic drugs administered in accordance with the analgesic 'ladder' described below. At the same time the following provisions should be applied:

(1)   First treat the cancer – try to arrange the possibility of radiotherapy, surgery or chemohormonal therapy. It is important to communicate with a specialist oncologist in order to plan therapy, particularly if the patient has lymphoma, seminoma or breast cancer (see Chapter 8).

(2)   If there is pain due to intestinal obstruction, palliative surgery should be considered as initial therapy (bypass, enterostomy, colostomy) (see Chapter 9).

(3)   If there is pain on movement of a part this requires immobilization. Vertebral collapse requires a rigid corset and external braces or splints. In cases of pain on movement due to the fracture of long bones or the spine, orthopaedic surgery should be considered.

(4)   If there is deafferentation pain this might be relieved by anticonvulsant drugs plus sympathetic block (see Chapter 7).

(5)   If there is localized severe pain which is inadequately relieved by drugs, refer to hospital for nerve block or neurosurgical treatment if possible (see Chapters 10, 11).

(6)   If there is nerve pressure pain use steroid drugs (see Chapter 7) or consider the possibility of decompression surgery (see Chapter 12).

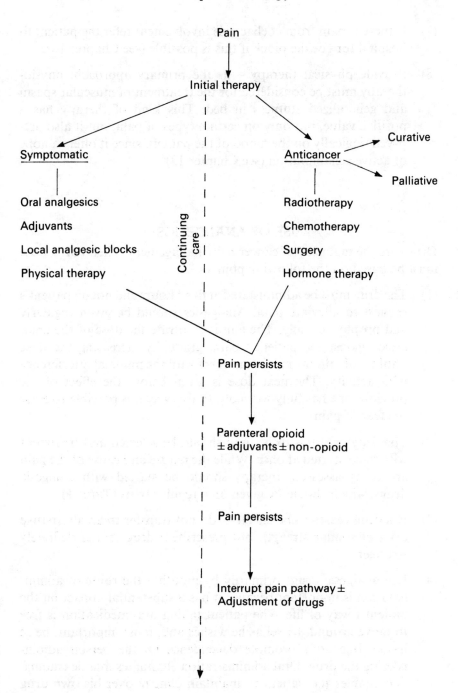

Figure 6 Flow chart – treatment of cancer pain

(7) If there is pain from coeliac axis involvement refer the patient to hospital for coeliac block if this is possible (see Chapter 10).

(8) Provide physical therapy – as the primary approach, physio-therapy must be considered for the treatment of muscular spasm and generalized stiffness in bed. This kind of therapy has a positive value, not only on certain types of pain, but it also acts psychologically on the mood of the patient, since it offers a hope of active rehabilitation (see Chapter 13).

USE OF ANALGESICS

Drugs are the mainstay of cancer pain management. Their correct use must be based on the following points.

(1) The drug must be administered at fixed hours and not on patient's request to alleviate pain. Analgesics should be given regularly and prophylactically. The aim is to titrate the dose of the analgesic against the patient's pain, gradually increasing the dose until we obtain the maximum relief with the minimal interference with activity. The next dose is given before the effect of the previous one has fully worn off. In this way it is possible to erase the fear of pain.

(2) The drug or drugs to be used should be selected and treatment with them started at once. While the nature and cause of the pain are being assessed, therapy should be started with analgesic drugs, which should be given on a regular basis (Table 1).

(3) If a drug ceases to be effective, do not transfer to an alternative drug of similar strength but prescribe a drug that is definitely stronger.

(4) Use analgesic drugs primarily by mouth – the route of admin-istration is important because it has a substantial impact on the patient's way of life. The patient taking oral medication is free to move around, travel as he wishes and, most important, be at home. Injections promote dependence on the person admin-istering the drug. Oral administration eliminates muscle trauma, and enables the patient to maintain control over his own drug administration.

(5) Use pure drugs, not compounds. With a compound an increase

Table 1   Basic drug list

Type	First choice	Alternatives
Non-opioids	aspirin	paracetamol (acetaminophen)
Weak opioids	codeine	dextropropoxyphene, oxymorphone
Strong opioids	morphine	methadone buprenorphine levorphanol standardized opium
Adjuvants		
Anticonvulsants	carbamazepine	phenytoin
Antidepressants	amitriptyline	clomipramine
Anxiolytics	diazepam	hydroxyzine
Corticosteroids	prednisolone	dexamethasone
Muscle relaxants	diazepam	baclofen
Psychotropics	chlorpromazine	haloperidol

in the dose of one drug will automatically increase the dose of the other whether it is necessary or not.

(6) Check interaction with any other substances (chemotherapeutic, hormonal, etc.) which the patient is receiving.

(7) Control side-effects.

(8) Learn how to use a few drugs well. The three basic analgesics are aspirin, codeine and morphine. Certain adjuvant drugs can also be helpful in certain specific cases. Learn to be familiar with one or two alternatives of each type of agent for use in patients who cannot tolerate the first choice drug. Your basic analgesic ladder, with alternatives, should include no more than nine or ten drugs in total. It is better to use and understand a few drugs well than to have a slight acquaintance with a large number.

Analgesics should be administered according to a sequential scale. The analgesic ladder is as shown in Figure 7.

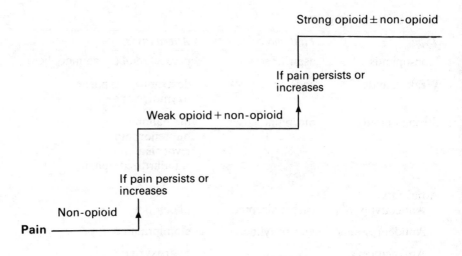

Figure 7   Analgesic 'ladder'

1st step

Use non-opioid drugs, such as aspirin or others of the antirheumatic drugs and alternatively paracetamol. These drugs should also be used particularly where there is intense pain due to nociception from the periosteum (bone pain), from the muscular fasciae, from the sub-cutaneous tissue or from a serous membrane, such as the pleura or the peritoneum, where there is no involvement of the large nervous trunks. Continuous administration of these substances can produce a reduction in the pain even during the first 24 hours.

Association with adjuvants such as tricyclic antidepressants, or anxiolytics to increase sleep can add to the analgesic effect. This form of treatment should be continued as long as it is helpful.

Passing on to the 2nd step can be necessary for the following reasons:

(1)   Inefficacy of the non-opioid drug after at least 24/48 hours.

(2)   Presence of side-effects from the drugs (example: gastritis, ulcer, haemorrhagic syndromes, etc.) which contraindicate their use.

2nd step

Use codeine or dextropropoxyphene. One of these drugs should be added to the aspirin or paracetamol immediately that the latter become inadequate. Adjuvant drugs should be added if symptoms such as insomnia, depression or anxiety are present (see Chapter 7).

If, despite the use of adequate doses of these drugs, the pain persists for more than 24–48 hours there should be no hesitation in starting the 3rd step.

3rd step

Administer opioid analgesics. As a first choice morphine should be used and as a second choice, methadone, in addition to the NSAID drug. In this way both central and peripheral actions on pain are obtained. The combination with adjuvant drugs can be useful in increasing the number of hours of sleep, especially if administered with anxiolytics or antidepressants. However, once strong opioids are being used the patient must be closely monitored, since the problems of titrating dosage and of the side-effects come into play. These problems can be overcome only by constant supervision.

In some clinical situations some of the adjuvant substances can be used alone to control pain; for example, steroids such as dexamethasone in pain caused by raised intracranial pressure or intraspinal compression, and the tricyclic antidepressants and anticonvulsants in some cases of pain caused by deafferentation (e.g. peripheral nerve injury, phantom limb, postherpetic neuralgia). In these conditions opioids are not very effective.

If due to weakness, nausea or vomiting the patient cannot swallow medication, you should resort to subcutaneous or intramuscular administration of analgesics or the sublingual or rectal route should be employed. If this type of administration is used, remember the difference in dosage which exists between the different ways of administering these drugs (see Chapter 7).

USE OF NEURODESTRUCTIVE THERAPIES

When pain is not being controlled by any of the above-mentioned drugs, or if medication does reduce the pain, but seriously worsens the 'quality of life' of the patient, we should consider neurodestructive procedures to the pain pathways if these are available.

It must be remembered that neurodestructive operations may interfere with some of the nervous functions of the part involved.

Neurolesion must have the following characteristics:

(1) It must be highly selective on the sensory pathway.

(2) It must not create new functional deficits in addition to the
     existing ones.

(3) It must not be carried out on a pre-existing neurolesion.

(4) It must not be painful.

(5) Above all, the procedure and its possible side-effects must be
     accepted by the patient.

All these interventions (including phenol or alcohol rhizotomy, and
neurosurgical interventions) must be performed in a hospital with
adequate facilities and expertise. These interventions can not only
reduce the pain, but also diminish, or abolish, for more or less long
periods of time, the use of analgesic drugs.

Evaluation of the aspects of the quality of life of the patient (performance status and persistent pain) should be important factors in
the choice of these treatments.

If the pain returns after surgery the administration of analgesics
should be recommenced. Pain control should be maintained until the
death of the patient.

CONTINUING CARE

Successful evaluation and treatment of pain in cancer patients implies
continuity of care from diagnosis onwards. There is no single approach
that offers consistently excellent results. It is crucial to reassure the
patients that pain relief will be provided throughout their illness to
allow them to function at a level that they choose and to die relatively
pain-free.

Continuous monitoring of the patient becomes essential from the
time that he requires potent opioids to relieve his pain (3rd step of the
analgesic ladder). New pains can appear and old pain can re-emerge.
As well as the control of physical pain, one must control all the other
symptoms, such as nausea, vomiting, decubitus ulcers, oral cavity or
bladder problems, etc. (see Chapter 12).

The major goals of continuing care are to provide the patient with:

(1) Relief from pain and other distressing symptoms, either in hospital or in his home.

(2) Psychological and social care.

(3) A support system to help him live as actively as possible in the face of impending death.

(4) Psychological care for the family during the illness and in bereavement.

(5) The family must be taught how they can help with the care of the patient.

There are a number of different ways in which this degree of care can be achieved.

One method is to have a small hospital or home (hospice) devoted entirely to continuing terminal care. Many hospices provide both inpatient and outpatient/home care. This is not always possible, and there are a variety of other approaches. Variations include a Symptom Control or Hospice Team functioning as a multidisciplinary consultation and support group within a general hospital, and Home Care alone. Moreover, inpatient units fall into two categories: another is a palliative care unit within or adjacent to a general hospital.

In this programme, specialist nurses working in the community help to achieve drug compliance; monitor for unacceptable drug side-effects and help to optimize analgesic, laxative, antiemetic and night sedative dosage between outpatient appointments. This therapeutic activity is, in one sense, comparable to the hospital nurse's freedom to administer 'as required' drugs. Liaison with the hospital doctor and with the family doctor is clearly important, indeed imperative. As with other specialist nurses (and physiotherapists), their knowledge is often invaluable in providing needed additional support, both psychosocial and practical.

Outpatient continuing care may demand very intensive specialist nurse involvement if initial problems are to be overcome, symptoms controlled and admission to hospital avoided. She should know not only how to manage pain problems but also how to care for other clinical problems (e.g. stoma care) (see Chapter 12). At other times, the specialist nurse acts simply as adviser to the primary community nurses. In addition, when appropriate, the nurse offers support to families in bereavement.

Home care

Most continuing care is home based. However, for those with more severe symptoms and those with little or no family support it may be better if they can be admitted to a hospital which offers continuing care facilities. It is very difficult to care adequately at home for the patient who is severely dyspnoeic or has gastrointestinal obstruction, or for the confused, bedfast octogenarian living alone. In most patients, particularly in those with few troublesome symptoms and adequate support from family and neighbours, home care is a realistic option that should be actively encouraged.

In many situations the patient, caring family member or close friend, community nurse and physician will constitute an adequate team.

The way you arrange your continuing care service will depend upon the conditions and circumstances of your country and your part of the country. However, whichever way you find the most effective, it is important that the following provisions are carried out:

Physician-directed service

A physician, preferably based in a hospital, should be in total charge of the organization and management of the continuing care programme. This doctor should ideally be able to co-ordinate with the various specialists mentioned in this book. He should try to acquire a good knowledge of pharmacology and psychosocial care.

Co-ordination of home and hospice care

This service must be organized in such a way that patients on home care can if possible be admitted to hospital temporarily when this is necessary and that hospitalized patients can be sent home with continuing close supervision. This supervision can be organized by the family, periodically reporting the patient's clinical condition to the doctor. In general the patient and family should be involved in the treatment as much as possible. Alternatively, the reports can be made by a specialist nurse who visits the patient at least once or twice a week.

Utilization of volunteers

Some people living in the community, regardless of class or educational standard, are willing to help to look after suffering individuals. These volunteers can be extremely helpful if they are properly trained by the doctor and nurse. At the request of the specialist nurse the volunteers can visit the patient and give social and psychological support both to him and his family.

Recommended reading

1. Bonica, J.J. and Ventafridda, V. (eds.) (1979). *Advances in Pain Research and Therapy*. Vol. 2. (New York: Raven Press).
2. Twycross, R.G. and Lack, S.A. (1984). *Therapeutics in Terminal Care*. (London: Pitman).
3. *Cancer Pain Relief* (1986) (Geneva: WHO)

7

Drug Therapy

Based on WHO's *Cancer Pain Relief**

I – Non-opioid Drugs

Aspirin and paracetamol (acetominophen) are the commonly available non-opioid analgesics for the management of mild to moderate pain (Table 2). These compounds have peripheral mechanisms of action. Aspirin is especially beneficial in metastatic bone pain where commonly there is a high local concentration of prostaglandin produced by the tumour cells. Aspirin provides pain relief by blocking prostaglandin biosynthesis; it also has anti-inflammatory and antipyretic effects. In patients with bone pain who are intolerant of aspirin, one

Table 2 Non-opioid drugs

Drug	Suggested dosage	Side-effects
Aspirin	250–1000 mg every 4–6 hours	Gastrointestinal disturbance + + Faecal blood loss + +

Note: The gastric side-effects may be reduced if taken with milk, on a full stomach, or with antacids. The administration of more than 4 g/day produces an increase in side-effects without proportionate increased pain relief.

Paracetamol	500–1000 mg every 4–6 hours	Liver toxicity

Note: Use with caution in patients with liver damage. The total dose per day should be 4–6 g

* See page 197.

of the non-steroidal anti-inflammatory drugs (NSAID) commonly used in arthritic conditions should be considered (e.g. ibuprofen, naproxen, diclofenac, indomethacin). Repeat doses of NSAID give a plateau effect beyond which increasing amounts produce little or no additional relief.

Aspirin-like analgesics may also be effective in relieving pain caused by: (1) mechanical distension of periosteum; (2) mechanical compression of tendon, muscle or subcutaneous tissue; and (3) mechanical compression of pleura or peritoneum.

ADMINISTRATION OF ASPIRIN

Aspirin is normally administered in tablet form and should be taken after meals or with a glass of milk. Soluble preparations (e.g. dispersible and buffered aspirin) are available in some countries for patients with dysphagia. These are also less irritant to the stomach. Aspirin suppositories are available in some countries.

Patients unable to take aspirin, but who would benefit from the use of an anti-inflammatory drug, may well tolerate one of the alternative NSAID preparations. Some of these need to be taken only once or twice a day.

Aspirin is readily absorbed from the upper gastrointestinal tract. After absorption its main action is at the site of the pain. Several days administration is necessary to achieve maximum relief.

SIDE-EFFECTS OF ASPIRIN AND NSAID

Toxic manifestations are related to the concentration of the free drug which varies inversely with the plasma albumin concentration. Hypoalbuminaemic patients are therefore more susceptible to toxic manifestations. Hence the drug should be given with caution to undernourished patients and those with far advanced cancer, many of whom come into this category.

Gastrointestinal effects

These are the most important side-effects. Aspirin may damage the gastric mucosa causing erosive gastritis and gastric haemorrhage. Symptoms are heartburn, dyspepsia, nausea, and vomiting; objective signs are blood loss in faeces and anaemia. These may be exacerbated by concomitant cancer chemotherapy. Patients who continue to have gastric intolerance to aspirin should be given a suitable antacid.

Effects on haemostasis and coagulation

The NSAID cause inhibition of platelet aggregation which leads to prolongation of bleeding time. In contrast to paracetamol, aspirin can cause irreversible effects on platelets; these effects disappear only when new platelets are formed.

Tinnitus

This is a common early warning symptom of toxic effect with aspirin.

Hypersensitivity

The clinical manifestations of this relatively rare syndrome may develop within minutes of drug ingestion. They range from vasomotor rhinitis with profuse watery secretion, angioneurotic oedema, urticaria, and bronchial asthma to laryngeal oedema and bronchoconstriction, hypotension, shock, loss of consciousness, and complete vasomotor collapse. This reaction may occur in response to small amounts of aspirin.

PARACETAMOL

In patients with non-bony pain who are intolerant of aspirin, paracetamol is the alternative drug of choice.

Paracetamol (acetaminophen) is a synthetic non-opioid analgesic. Like aspirin, it is antipyretic but in contrast to aspirin, it normally has no anti-inflammatory effect. As an analgesic it acts peripherally. It is mainly absorbed from the small intestine; 25% of subjects are slow absorbers. Drugs that delay gastric emptying delay the absorption of paracetamol. The recommended dosage is 500-1000 mg every 4–6 hours. Within this range, paracetamol is equipotent with aspirin.

Paracetamol is mostly excreted in the urine. It should be used with caution in patients with liver disease. The total dose recommended is 4–6 g per day.

A regular intake of 2 g of paracetamol per day may result in an increase in thrombotest time, necessitating a reduction in the dose of coumarin anticoagulants if these are given concurrently.

The other main distinguishing features of paracetamol are: (a) it can be taken by those hypersensitive to aspirin; (b) it is well tolerated by patients with peptic ulcer; (c) it does not affect plasma uric acid concentration; (d) it has no effect on platelet function; and (e) side-effects are minor and minimal.

Serious toxicity does not occur when paracetamol is used in therapeutic doses, that is, up to 1 g every 4 hours.

Paracetamol can be obtained as an elixir, a syrup, or a solution but it is normally administered as a tablet.

RECOMMENDATIONS FOR THE USE OF NON-OPIOID ANALGESICS

(1) Enquire if the patient tolerates aspirin and aspirin-like compounds to avoid allergic phenomena.

(2) Non-opioid analgesic should be used regularly by the clock in order to avoid pain recurrence.

(3) An adequate amount of the drug should be administered. However, these drugs have ceiling effects and doses above those recommended will not give additional analgesia

(4) Non-opioid analgesics may be used alone or in combination with psychotropic or opioid drugs.

(5) Side-effects should be looked out for as described above; if they occur, change to an alternative non-opioid. If the side-effects are uncontrollable, consider administration of a weak opioid.

When a non-opioid drug, with or without adjuvants, no longer controls the pain a weak opioid analgesic should be combined with the non-opioid analgesic.

II – Opioid Drugs

WEAK OPIOID ANALGESICS

The most important weak opioids are codeine and dextro-propoxyphene. Codeine is to be preferred, but dextropropoxyphene is a useful alternative. These drugs are taken by mouth. Constipation is the main side-effect and can be prevented by the use of laxatives (e.g. senna). Nausea and vomiting also may occur. Physical dependence and tolerance may occur but are not a common problem when these drugs are used in pain management.

Codeine

30 mg of codeine is approximately equianalgesic to 650 mg of aspirin when taken by mouth. Codeine is readily absorbed when taken orally.

When the two drugs are combined, the analgesic effect equals or exceeds that of 60 mg codeine. Codeine may, of course, be used alone (average dose 30–80 mg 4-hourly).

The suggested oral dosage of codeine phosphate in association with aspirin or paracetamol is: 30–130 mg codeine (average 60–80 mg) with 500 mg of paracetamol or 250–500 mg of aspirin every 4–6 hours.

Dextropropoxyphene

With repeated oral administration every 6 hours, a steady state is reached after 2–3 days but it is cumulative in continued repeated dosage. High doses occasionally produce central nervous system effects such as hallucination, confusion and convulsions.

Suggested oral dosage is 60 mg every 4 hours. Dextropropoxyphene in combination with aspirin 250–600 mg or paracetamol 500 mg provides an analgesic effect superior to that of each compound taken individually.

The drug is available as propoxyphene hydrochloride and propoxyphene napsylate; 100 mg of napsylate is equivalent to 65 mg of hydrochloride.

When the pain is no longer controlled by a weak opioid combined with aspirin or paracetamol (and if necessary an adjuvant), the patient should be started on a strong opioid.

STRONG OPIOID ANALGESICS

General considerations

The strong opioid analgesics are the mainstay of therapy of moderate and severe cancer pain because when properly used, they provide effective pain relief in most patients. The safe and rational use of opioid analgesics must be based on an understanding of their clinical pharmacology.

The use of strong opioid analgesics is associated with development of tolerance and sometimes physical dependence. These are normal pharmacological responses to their chronic use. *Physical dependence* is characterized by withdrawal symptoms if treatment is stopped abruptly. *Tolerance* is characterized by decreasing efficacy with repeated administration and it may require an increase of the dose to maintain the analgesic effect, but the drug will still be effective.

Psychological dependence is a behavioural pattern of drug abuse characterized by drug craving and overwhelming involvement for the procurement of the drug. Undue concern about psychological dependence ('addiction') has caused doctors and nurses to use opioids in inadequate doses. Wide clinical experience has shown that psychological dependence rarely, if ever, occurs in cancer patients receiving opioid analgesics for chronic pain. In cancer patients, pain is an important symptom that can and must be treated.

Even after chronic use oral morphine can be discontinued if the cause of pain is treated successfully with anticancer therapy (e.g. radiotherapy or chemotherapy). The dose should be decreased gradually, possibly over a period of 3 or more weeks. In this way withdrawal symptoms are avoided.

Many factors must be considered if strong opioids are to be used effectively. These include age, nutritional status, extent of disease and, in particular, involvement of the liver and the kidneys. In the elderly, lower initial doses should be used because of changes in the pharmacodynamics of the drugs and increased response. Malnutrition gives rise to changes in body composition and function and also necessitates lower initial doses. Since the response of each patient varies, it is necessary to select the most appropriate drug and administer it in an individualized dose and by the simplest route. Oral administration is preferable, but in certain situations these drugs have to be administered sublingually, rectally, or parenterally.

The standard recommended dose must be adjusted according to individual need. This depends on the intensity of the pain, prior analgesic medication and the disposition of the drug. The latter may be altered by intercurrent diseases when it may be necessary to start with lower initial doses and increase or decrease the dose according to the patient's needs.

Most strong opioid analgesics are metabolized primarily in the liver, and their elimination is therefore dependent on liver function. Liver dysfunction occurs with various tropical diseases. Involvement of the liver is not a contraindication to the use of opioids; in contrast to high doses of paracetamol and some of the adjuvant drugs, the opioid analgesics are not known to be hepatotoxic. However, care should be exercised when using these drugs in patients with liver dysfunction. In patients with liver cirrhosis the oral bioavailability (fraction of oral dose reaching the systemic circulation) has been shown to be increased for pethidine (and for dextropropoxyphene). The clearance (volume of blood cleared in unit time) is decreased and the duration of action of the drugs is therefore increased. This may lead to accentuated effects and side-effects at comparatively low doses.

With few exceptions the metabolites of most drugs are excreted by the kidneys. Therefore, renal dysfunction leads to accumulation of metabolites some of which may cause myoclonus and seizures at high concentrations. Opioids are therefore contraindicated in patients with severe renal dysfunction.

Some liver and kidney diseases are associated with low albumin levels, which may decrease the plasma protein binding and hence increase the sensitivity to the drug (including aspirin). Severe degrees of malnutrition also may alter the response and disposition of these drugs. In such patients it is necessary to use opioids with great care. Malnutrition is not, however, a contraindication to their use.

Use of strong opioid analgesics

Opioid analgesics must be administered in an acceptable form. The oral route is the best because it spares the patient the discomfort of injections and maintains his independence since he does not have to rely on someone else for his next dose.

Morphine by mouth – Morphine can be administered as a simple aqueous solution of morphine sulphate (or hydrochloride) in a range of strengths (e.g. morphine sulphate 1–20 mg/ml). An antimicrobial preservative is necessary, particularly in hotter climates. The taste is bitter and some patients prefer to take the medicine with a drink to mask the taste. The solution should be stored in a dark bottle which should be kept in a cool place and not exposed to direct sunlight. Morphine can also be made up in a syrup (see Appendix).

Sustained release morphine tablets are available in some countries in strengths varying from 10 to 100 mg. The most widely available strength is 30 mg. These tablets need to be given only every 8–12 hours. With long-acting agents the titration of the initial dose tends to be more difficult.

The effective analgesic dose of morphine varies considerably and ranges from as little as 5 mg to more than 200 mg. Many patients are satisfactorily controlled in doses of between 5 and 30 mg every 4 hours. However, dosage varies greatly in different patients because of wide individual variations in oral bioavailability of the drug and the appropriate dose is the one that works. The drug must be given by the clock (e.g. every 4 hours) and not only when the patient complains of pain. The use of morphine is dictated by intensity of pain and not by brevity of prognosis.

Instruction to the patient

Emphasize the need for regular administration every 4 hours. The first and last dose of the day are 'anchored' to the patient's waking and bedtimes. The best additional times during the day are generally 10 a.m., 2 p.m. and 6 p.m. At these intervals there is an optimal balance between duration of analgesic effect and severity of side-effects. Ideally, the patient's drug regimen should be written out in full for the patient and his family to work from, including times to be taken, names of drugs, reason for use (e.g. 'for pain', 'for bowels') and dose (x ml, y tablets). The patient should be warned about possible initial side-effects.

Choice of starting dose

The initial dose of morphine sulphate depends mainly on the patient's previous medication. For those previously receiving a weak opioid (codeine, dextropropoxyphene), a starting dose of 5 mg may be adequate, though many require 10 mg, and occasionally more.

If the patient is extremely somnolent after the first dose and is pain free, the second dose should be reduced by 50%. If, after 24 hours on the medication there is insufficient analgesia, the starting dose should be increased by 50%. Meanwhile, the starting dose can be repeated more frequently than 4-hourly to avoid excessive pain.

The patient must be reassessed after 24 and 72 hours, preferably by the doctor. If pain relief is not adequate with the drug being given or it causes unacceptable side-effects, another strong opioid drug should be tried. Sometimes the patient has a type of pain unresponsive to opioids, in which case non-drug measures (e.g. nerve blocks) should be considered, if available. Occasionally there is a marked psychological component to the pain and an anxiolytic or antidepressant may be indicated. If no therapy produces pain relief, a search should be initiated for other factors contributing to the pain complaint.

Night-time

The drug should be given through the night or in a larger dose at bedtime to sustain the plasma level of the drug in an effective range. With a 50% or a 100% increase in dose at bedtime, many patients do not need a middle-of-the-night dose.

Patients requiring doses of 60 mg or more of morphine usually need a middle-of-the-night dose to avoid waking in pain in the later part of the night.

Control of unwanted effects
Nausea

If the patient is nauseated at the time of commencing treatment, prescribe an antiemetic concurrently, such as prochlorperazine 5–10 mg 8-hourly increasing to 4-hourly, or metaclopramide 10 mg 8-hourly, increasing to 4-hourly. Haloperidol 1–2 mg daily is a useful alternative (see Chapter 12).

If the patient is vomiting, the antiemetic will need to be given intramuscularly, possibly for up to 2 days. If the patient is not nauseated, it is generally advisable to issue a 4-day supply of an antiemetic for the patient to use prophylactically or as required, in order to avoid initial nausea or vomiting.

Drowsiness, dizziness, unsteadiness

Warn the patient about initial drowsiness etc., but emphasize that these will clear up after 3–5 days on a constant dose.

Confusion

Warn older patients that they may become muddled at times during the first few days, but to persevere with the medication.

Constipation

Almost all patients become constipated unless they have a colostomy or steatorrhoea. A laxative should be prescribed when morphine is started, preferably given at night. Dietary measures also should be taken if possible. The control of constipation may be more difficult than the control of pain (see Chapter 12). For most patients, the regular use of senna counteracts the constipation. Like morphine, the dose has to be titrated for each patient until a satisfactory result is achieved. Two tablets of standardized senna at bedtime is the usual starting dose, increasing to two tablets 2–3 times a day, or more if necessary. Some patients may require a second or alternative laxative. If the patient is severely constipated when an opioid is first prescribed, the use of suppositories or an enema is an important first step.

Morphine intolerance

A minority of patients have delayed gastric emptying causing persistent intermittent vomiting; a few experience marked persistent sedation. On rare occasions, a patient experiences psychotic symptoms, or symptoms relating to histamine release (pruritus, bronchoconstriction). These patients should be given an alternative strong opioid analgesic.

Alternative strong opioid analgesics

For most patients requiring a strong opioid, morphine is both efficacious and acceptable and it is the drug of choice. If a patient appears to have persistent intolerance to morphine, an alternative that is chemically distinct should be used in the hope that this does not cause the unwanted effect.

Methadone

Methadone is a synthetic narcotic analgesic whose effects are generally similar to those of morphine and is absorbed well from all routes of administration. Orally it is about one half to three quarters as potent as by subcutaneous or intramuscular injection. Maximum analgesia and side-effects produced by methadone are not achieved until 4–14 days after commencement. Given in a single dose, methadone is marginally more potent than morphine but, in repeated dosage, it is several times more potent. Its effective analgesic range is the same as that of morphine. It is generally longer acting than morphine, useful analgesia lasting some 6–8 hours. The suggested dosage is 5–10 mg every 6 hours by mouth for the first 3 days after which the dose is given every 8–12 hours or even longer. If necessary methadone can be administered by injection.

Methadone, like morphine, has no obvious ceiling effect. Compared to morphine, greater care needs to be exercised when using methadone, particularly at first until a patient's response to it has been fully evaluated. Extra care should be taken when psychotropic drugs are being administered concurrently.

Methadone accumulates in the blood on repeated dosage. It should therefore not be used: (1) in the elderly or demented; (2) in those with confusional symptoms; (3) in patients with significant respiratory, hepatic or renal dysfunction.

Rifampicin, an antituberculous antibiotic, speeds up methadone metabolism and sometimes precipitates withdrawal symptoms.

Pethidine

Pethidine (meperidine) is a synthetic opioid analgesic. Its effects are generally similar to those of morphine but it is only about one eighth as potent as morphine. It also has atropine-like effects. It is about one third as potent by mouth as by subcutaneous or intramuscular injection. It may not relieve such severe pain as morphine, but in higher doses it is considerably more effective than codeine. It is generally shorter acting than morphine, useful analgesia lasting 3–4 hours.

Pethidine is not a complete alternative to morphine. It may need to be given every 3 hours in patients with severe cancer pain because of its shorter duration of action. Equianalgesic doses of pethidine and morphine produce a similar incidence of side-effects such as vomiting or depression of the respiratory centre. The recommended dose is 50–100 mg every 3–4 hours.

With pethidine, the incidence of unwanted central nervous system (CNS) effects (i.e. tremor, twitching, agitation and convulsions) increases considerably at doses above 200 mg 3-hourly. Pethidine should not be given to patients with impaired renal function because of the increased likelihood of CNS side-effects. Phenobarbitone and chlorpromazine increase the toxicity of pethidine.

Buprenorphine

Buprenorphine is a strong opioid analgesic and is a representative of a group of opioid drugs called *mixed agonist-antagonists*. They should not be used with other opioid analgesics as they may reverse analgesia. Buprenorphine has a ceiling effect; it is not a complete alternative to morphine. Morphine-like effects are maximal at a dose of about 1 mg intramuscularly. Onset of action arises in about 30 min, and peak effect comes after 3 hours (morphine 1–2 hours). The duration of useful effect is 6–9 hours (morphine 4–5 hours). Most patients are satisfactorily controlled on an 8-hourly regimen. It should be taken *sublingually*.

Subjective and psychological effects are generally similar to those of morphine but, unlike morphine, increasing the dosage leads to dysphoria. Compared with orally administered morphine, sublingual buprenorphine is some 60–80 times more potent (i.e. the dose of buprenorphine is 1/60–1/80 that of morphine). In patients whose pain is no longer controlled by buprenorphine, a change should be made to oral morphine sulphate. The initial starting dose of morphine in this circumstance is determined by multiplying by 100 the previously administered total daily dose of buprenorphine. This total daily dose should be converted to a convenient 4-hourly regimen of morphine. The dependence liability of buprenorphine is less than that of codeine.

Other strong opioids

In some countries, some of the above opioids may not be available but other strong opioids can be obtained. Most will substitute for oral morphine and the following should be satisfactory.

Standardized opium – This is virtually diluted morphine; the morphine content varies from country to country but is usually 10% of the weight of opium powder. The doctor should determine the morphine content in his country. In some countries it is manufactured in a fixed dose combination tablet with aspirin.

Levorphanol – It is five times more potent than oral morphine. It provides relief for 4–6 hours. Like methadone, it may accumulate in the blood and may produce sedation with repeated doses. The normal starting dose is 2–4 mg by mouth or 1–2 mg i.m.

ALTERNATIVE ROUTES OF ADMINISTERING OPIOIDS

Rectal administration

Morphine may be given per rectum; this is as effective as by mouth. This route may be useful in patients who are vomiting or too ill to take oral medication. In some countries, suppositories are available in strengths ranging from 10 to 60 mg. When suppositories are not available, it is possible to administer morphine by rectal enema, the dose being contained in 10–20 ml of water. Opium can also be given per rectum.

Subcutaneous or intramuscular injection

If the patient is unable to take oral or rectal opioid analgesics, the subcutaneous or intramuscular route should be used. Morphine, methadone, and buprenorphine may be given subcutaneously; pethidine must be given by deep intramuscular injection. The parenteral dose of morphine will be about one third to one half of the previously satisfactory oral dose. In the case of methadone, the oral dose should be halved; with buprenorphine, the oral dose is used.

Opium and levorphanol can also be administered parenterally. When changing from the oral to the parenteral route, it may be necessary to retitrate the dose of analgesic.

Epidural and intrathecal administration

These new methods of administration have been developed to provide selective pain relief with minimal side-effects. They require specific expertise for catheter placement and specialized equipment and close supervision. Although effective, their role in cancer pain management remains controversial (see Recommended reading).

III – Adjuvant Drugs

GENERAL CONSIDERATIONS

Adjuvant drugs are compounds of various chemical structure which are used for cancer pain management in one of two ways:

(1) To treat specific types of pain which do not respond to morphine (Table 3).

(2) To ameliorate other symptoms that commonly occur in cancer patients (Table 4).

Table 3 Types of pain relatively unresponsive to morphine

Tension headache
Postherpetic neuralgia
Dysaesthesia
Stabbing pain
Visceral pain
Muscle spasm
Nerve compression
Activity precipitated
Decubitus (superficial component)
Deafferentation

Table 4 Adjuvant drugs

Class	Analgesic effect	Antidepressant effect	Anxiolytic effect	Muscle relaxant	Antiemetic	Anticonfusional
Anticonvulsants						
carbamazepine	a					
phenytoin	a					
Psychotropic						
prochlorperazine					+	
chlorpromazine			+	(+)	+	
haloperidol			+		+	+
hydroxyzine	+		+			
diazepam			+	+		
amitriptyline	b	+	(+)			
Corticosteroids						
prednisolone	c	(+)				
dexamethasone	c	(+)				

a Often of benefit in lancinating (shooting, stabbing) pain
b Often of benefit in dysaesthetic (superficial burning) pain
c Often of use in nerve compression, spinal cord compression, raised intracranial pressure

Any attempt to develop guidelines for the use of these drugs in cancer pain management must be prefaced by certain provisions:

(1) To enhance analgesia or to treat side-effects with these drugs requires careful assessment of the patient's symptoms and clinical signs.

(2) Adjuvant drugs should not be prescribed routinely. The choice of drug is always dictated by the need of the individual patient. The drugs used to treat specific types of pain include anticonvulsants, antidepressants and corticosteroids. The drugs used to ameliorate symptoms include neuroleptics, anxiolytics and antidepressants (Table 5).

Table 5 Adjuvants for specific pain syndromes

Type of pain	Adjuvant indicated
Bone pain	Aspirin or NSAID
Raised intracranial pressure	Corticosteroids
Nerve pressure pain	Corticosteroids, anticonvulsants
Nerve destruction pain (deafferentation)	Antidepressants, anticonvulsants
Superficial dysaesthetic pain	Antidepressants
Intermittent stabbing pain	Anticonvulsants
Gastric distension pain	Metoclopramide
Rectal/bladder tenesmus pain	Chlorpromazine
Muscle spasm pain	Diazepam
Pain and depression	Tricyclic antidepresant (avoid benzodiazepine)
Pain and anxiety	Benzodiazepine or phenothiazine

In ill and malnourished cancer patients, the concurrent use of two drugs that act on the central nervous system (e.g. morphine and a psychotropic drug or two psychotropic drugs) is likely to produce a greater sedative effect than in other circumstances. In cancer pain patients, the starting doses of psychotropic drugs are usually less than in physically healthy patients.

ANTICONVULSANTS

Carbamazepine and phenytoin are drugs whose mechanisms of action include the suppression of spontaneous neuronal firing. They have been used effectively in the management of specific neurological pain such as trigeminal neuralgia. In cancer, they are useful in the management of the stabbing component of deafferentation pain.

The initial dose of *carbamazepine* is 100 mg a day, increasing by 100 mg every 3–4 days if necessary, to a maximum dose of 400 mg or occasionally 500–600 mg. The major side-effects include nausea, vomiting, ataxia, dizziness, lethargy and confusion. These can be minimized by slow upward titration of dose at the start of medication and by close monitoring. Cancer patients are at a greater risk of developing leukopaenia if they have recently received chemotherapy. The dose of *phenytoin* should commence at 100 mg a day and be increased gradually by 25–50 mg increments to a total dose of not more than 300 mg per day. A steady state is achieved after 1–2 weeks. The side-effects are similar to those described for carbamazepine; they are usually mild and rarely interfere with therapy.

ANTIDEPRESSANTS

Antidepressants are used to relieve the dysaesthetic pain of deafferentation. In this situation, antidepressants – notably amitriptyline – produce analgesic effects at doses below those used to treat depression. Amitriptyline also has a hypnotic effect which helps to improve the patient's sleeping pattern.

In cancer patients with pain, antidepressants are also used to treat concurrent depression which occurs in up to 25% of cancer patients.

The starting dose of amitriptyline varies from 10 to 25 mg given in a single dose at bedtime. A slow increase to 50–75 mg per day is usually associated with improvement in the deafferentiation pain, and improvement in sleep. In patients with major depression, daily doses of up to 150–200 mg may be required. Side-effects include dry mouth, constipation, urinary retention, light-headedness and confusion. Rarely the drug may produce a hyperexcitable state. It is contra-indicated in patients with glaucoma.

CORTICOSTEROIDS

Corticosteroids may be used as adjuvants to analgesics, for mood enhancement and appetite stimulation. They have anti-inflammatory properties, and are useful in relieving pain associated with nerve compression, spinal cord compression, headache from raised intra-cranial pressure, and also bone pain. Both prednisolone and dexame-thasone are effective; 1 mg of dexamethasone is equivalent to 7 mg of prednisolone.

The dose is dependent on the clinical situation. For nerve com-pression pain, prednisolone 10 mg three times a day or dexamethasone 4 mg daily should be prescribed, dropping to a lower maintenance dose after 7–10 days. Occasionally a higher dose is necessary to achieve significant benefit. With raised intracranial pressure, an initial dose of dexamethasone 4 mg four times a day is appropriate. It may be possible to reduce this to a lower maintenance dose after 7–10 days. With cord compression, even higher doses have been used in some centres, up to 100 mg a day initially, tapering to 16 mg during radiation therapy.

Side-effects include oral candidiasis, oedema, dyspeptic symptoms, and, occasionally, gastrointestinal bleeding. Proximal myopathy, agi-tation, and hypomania may also occur. The incidence of gastro-intestinal side-effects may be increased if corticosteroids are used in conjunction with aspirin-like drugs.

NEUROLEPTICS

Chlorpromazine is not an analgesic and does not provide additive analgesia when combined with an opioid drug. It does have antianxiety effects and may be useful in reducing anxiety that is exacerbating pain. It also has antiemetic and antipsychotic properties. Side-effects include hypotension, blurred vision, dry mouth, tachycardia, urinary reten-tion, constipation and extrapyramidal effects. The dose is 10–25 mg orally every 4–8 hours.

Prochlorperazine is used as an antiemetic. The dose is 5–10 mg orally every 4–8 hours. Parenteral and suppository preparations are available.

Haloperidol is used most commonly in cancer for patients with an agitated confusional state. It is a more potent antiemetic than chlorpromazine and is less sedative with fewer antichollinergic and cardiovascular effects. 1 mg by mouth once or twice a day is the suggested starting dose. For the management of psychiatric symptoms, the doses are significantly higher – up to 10 mg two to three times a day.

ANXIOLYTICS

Diazepam is commonly used to manage acute anxiety and panic attacks. Anxiety is commonly seen in patients with pain, but it often diminishes once the pain is controlled. Diazepam does not provide additive analgesia when combined with an opioid drug. It is, however, useful in treating pain caused by muscle spasm. Side-effects include drowsiness, postural hypotension, and muscular hypotonia.

5–10 mg diazepam is the usual starting dose. It can be given by mouth, per rectum or parenterally. Maintenance treatment ranges from 2 to 10 mg at bedtime and up to 10 mg two or three times a day depending on individual needs.

Hydroxyzine has anxiolytic, antihistaminic, antispasmodic and antiemetic activity. When it is combined with morphine, additive analgesic effects occur. Side-effects include sedation, hyperexcitability and multifocal myoclonus. The dose is 10 mg three times a day to 25 mg 4-hourly, occasionally more.

Recommended reading

1. *Cancer Pain Relief* (1986) (Geneva: WHO)
2. Swerdlow, M. (ed.) (1986). *The Therapy of Pain*. 2nd Edn. (Lancaster: MTP Press).
3. Twycross, R. W. and Lack, S. A. (1983). *Symptom Control in Advanced Cancer: Pain Relief*. (London: Pitman).
4. Saunders, C. M. (ed.) (1984). *The Management of Terminal Disease*. (London: Edward Arnold).
5. Twycross, R. G. and Ventafridda, V. (eds.) (1980). *The Continuing Care of Terminal Cancer Patients*. (Oxford: Pergamon Press).

8

Chemotherapy and Radiotherapy for Cancer Pain

S. Monfardini and A. Scanni

INTRODUCTION

One approach to the control of cancer pain is to treat the cause of the pain by chemotherapy (including hormonal therapy), by radiation therapy or by surgery if this is possible. Some forms of cancer can now be cured; others can be helped by palliative oncological therapy. The goal of palliative treatment is to improve the quality of life for the patient and occasionally to prolong life. This chapter summarizes the current status of chemotherapy and radiation therapy in patients with cancer pain.

GENERAL PRINCIPLES

The general principles which the oncologist should follow in the use of antitumour therapy in patients with pain include:

(1) Understanding the nature of the pain and the extent of the patient's disease.

(2) Identifying the lesion(s) causing the pain and considering palliative therapy.

89

(3) Radiotherapy is used for localized lesions and chemotherapy or hormone therapy for diffuse disease.

(4) Antitumour therapies should be suited to the needs of the individual patient and appropriate combinations should be applied when indicated.

(5) Antitumour therapy will need to be modified if there is short life expectancy, organ failure, low performance status, or reduced patient compliance.

PAIN TREATMENT WITH CANCER CHEMOTHERAPY

Chemotherapy of cancer includes the use of a large number of important drugs (Table 6). These drugs are used either alone or more commonly in combination and in a wide range of schedules. Their clinical efficacy is well documented and a detailed review of each of these drugs and their clinical indications is not included here but can be found in the recommended reading.

Table 6 Main antineoplastic drugs used in clinical practice

Class	Drugs
Alkylating agents	Mechlorethamine, cyclophosphamide
Antimetabolites	Methotrexate, 5-fluorouracil
Plant alkaloids	Vincristine, vinblastine
Antibiotics	Adriamycin, bleomycin
Hormones	Antioestrogens, progestogens
Miscellaneous	Procarbazine, cis-platinum

Antitumour therapy can be effective in reducing pain when there is:

(1) destruction of tissue by tumour,

(2) rapid enlargement of viscera,

(3) local pressure and obstruction.

Cytotoxic drugs are helpful in chemosensitive tumours such as haematological malignancies, testicular carcinomas, small cell carcinoma of the lung and other solid tumours. Hormonal therapy is useful to palliate pain in endocrine-dependent tumours such as breast and prostatic carcinomas. In other clinical conditions, chemotherapy is only of limited value in relief of pain caused by advanced tumours because:

(1) Many solid tumours are not sufficiently responsive to current drug regimens.

(2) Pain usually develops in advanced stages of cancer when the tumour has become resistant to the first-line drug therapy.

(3) Pain is often produced by large tumour masses.

(4) Prior surgery and especially prior radiotherapy applied to the tumour site almost always prevent achievement of an effective drug concentration for a sufficiently long time.

Because cytotoxic drugs also damage normal cells, the toxic effect of these drugs directly limits their use and indirectly limits their efficacy. Cyclic chemotherapy is often the most effective way to reduce severe bone marrow suppression as well as oral and intestinal mucositis. Cumulative toxicity can be prevented in the majority of patients by discontinuing the administration of a given drug before the total risk dose is reached.

RADIATION THERAPY IN PATIENTS WITH CANCER-INDUCED PAIN

Radiotherapy arrests the division of both malignant and normal cells. Although the precise basic mechanism of the analgesic action of radiation therapy is not generally known, the most important beneficial effects result from: (a) reduction of pressure effects on nerves, brain or hollow organs; (b) reduction of infiltration; (c) disappearance of ulcerations; and (d) resolution of inflammatory reaction in the tumour and in its periphery.

Some tumour types are more sensitive than others (Table 7).

Pain caused by metastatic bone lesions usually responds to radiation; about 80–85% of cases achieve a good remission. In patients with advanced cancer with pain due to visceral lesions, radiation therapy is less effective.

Palliative radiotherapy uses the minimum dose and the minimum number of treatment sessions to relieve the pain. The side-effects that may occur must be balanced against the likely benefit.

Table 7   Radiosensitivity of tumour types

Highly radiosensitive tumours
Malignant lymphomas
Localized myelomas
Seminoma

Moderately radiosensitive tumours
Carcinoma of the skin
Epidermoid carcinomas of mucous membranes
Ewing's sarcoma
Adenocarcinomas (endometrium, breast, gastrointestinal tract)

Poorly radiosensitive tumours
Soft tissue sarcomas
Bone sarcomas
Malignant melanomas

The choice of radiotherapy dosage must be made according to the histology and the volume of the lesion responsible for the pain in order to secure a complete remission and to prevent an early relapse. The possibility of delivering the appropriate total radiation therapy dosage in a reduced time is clearly desirable. Palliation of bone metastases can be achieved in one session if high energy irradiation beams are available (See Recommended reading).

The causes of failure of radiotherapy are: (a) the poor responsivity to radiotherapy of certain types of tumours, such as malignant melanoma, mesothelioma, fibrosarcoma, leiomyosarcoma, and teratocarcinoma of the testis; (b) previous radiotherapy, at high doses; (c) tumours in the mouth, particularly the oral floor; (d) the presence of pathological fracture; (e) the formation of abscesses in the tumours; (f) the presence of neoplastic spread to bone segments contiguous with the primary tumour, with consequent destruction of the periosteum; (g) the presence of intense endosteal or periosteal reaction to the tumour; (h) technical errors in the irradiation.

CHEMO-RADIO-HORMONO-THERAPY OF PAIN FROM DIFFERENT TUMOURS AND CLINICAL SITUATIONS

Every malignant neoplasm may produce pain, but pain is particularly common in breast, lung, colon–rectum, oropharynx, prostate and testicular carcinomas, in leukaemias, lymphomas and in brain tumours.

Usually, localized lesions producing pain are initially treated with radiotherapy while diffused ones are treated with chemotherapy and/or hormonotherapy. However, medical and radiological approaches must always be considered as complementary modalities rather than competitive ones.

BREAST CANCER

Advanced breast cancer may cause pain by infiltration of the chest wall or by tumour ulceration. In these situations, chemotherapy and/or hormonotherapy will temporarily cause complete or partial remission in 50–70% of patients; the objective clinical response is almost always associated with a high degree of regression and even with disappearance of pain. Radiation therapy produces comparable clinical results.

With breast cancer the most common site of metastases and pain is in bone. These patients are not curable but they have a relatively high life expectancy and pain treatment is therefore of the utmost importance. Radiation therapy is effective mainly in osteolytic meta- stases which produce localized pain. With diffuse bone metastases, pain can be better controlled either by ablative hormonotherapy (ovariectomy, hypophysectomy, adrenalectomy) or by hormone therapy (progestogens, oestrogens, antioestrogens, androgens, amino- glutethimide). Chemotherapy can also be valuable in these particular clinical situations. Breast cancer can produce brain metastases and headache in which case whole brain irradiation represents the main treatment. Corticosteroids are usually administered together with the radiotherapy.

HEAD AND NECK CANCER

Headache and pharyngodynia are the most frequent types of pain with tumours in this region. Previous treatments often limit the pal- liative effects of radio- and chemotherapy. Considerable relief can be obtained with radiotherapy but chemotherapy can also be useful. Combined treatments can be given in full doses, because there is no additive effect on bone marrow. Sequential modalities are to be preferred in order to avoid oral mucositis from both radiotherapy and drug therapy.

BRAIN TUMOURS

In inoperable advanced primary brain tumours, radiotherapy is the main treatment and nitrosoureas (CCNU 130/mg/m^2 per os every 6 weeks) represent the main complementary drugs. Tension headache due to tumour expansion is relieved by the use of dexamethasone (24–16 mg, 8–4 times daily).

LUNG CANCER

Lung cancer can cause pain due to bone and brain metastases or by direct infiltration of nerves. In such cases, radiotherapy is useful. The therapeutic effects of chemotherapy are limited and transient in non-small-cell lung cancer, but in small-cell carcinomas, chemotherapy can induce objective remission. Pain caused by infiltration of the brachial plexus (Pancoast's syndrome) is a typical aspect of cancer growing in the apex of the lung. In this case, radiotherapy is preferable to chemotherapy.

PELVIC AND COLORECTAL CARCINOMA

These tumours which can produce a pain syndrome due to endopelvic diffusion have limited chemosensitivity.

Radiotherapy often represents the only means of palliative treatment. This treatment is frequently limited as the tumours may be less radioresponsive (adenocarcinoma) and diffuse.

PROSTATIC CANCER

In prostatic cancer, pain is essentially produced by osteolytic or osteoblastic (bone thickening) bone metastases. This tumour, as well as breast cancer, may be hormonodependent. Rapid pain relief can sometimes be induced by orchidectomy or oestrogens. Radiotherapy is less effective against pain produced by osteoblastic metastases and here chemotherapy can be useful.

TESTICULAR CANCER

Testicular cancer is usually responsive to chemotherapy and radiotherapy. It can produce lumbar pain when retroperitoneal lymph node metastases reach considerable dimensions. In this far advanced stage, metastases are unfortunately less responsive to chemotherapy. Testicular teratomas are less radiosensitive than seminomas.

ACUTE LEUKAEMIA

Diffuse pain in bone and joints, due to periosteal spread at the beginning of the disease can resemble a rheumatic syndrome. Appropriate polychemotherapy can induce a remission of disease and disappearance of pain. Radiotherapy can help, however, when symptoms are localized and non-responsive to chemotherapy.

Headache, due to meningeal infiltration, can be controlled, in almost all patients, by whole central nervous system irradiation and intrathecal infusion of methotrexate.

The medical oncologist and the radiotherapist know very well the value of an active attitude toward a pain inducing disease. On the other hand, the tendency towards an aggressive approach should be tempered by the consideration of those factors which may limit anticancer treatment in the patient with advanced cancer. Short life expectancy, low performance status, organ failure (pulmonary, renal or hepatic), lack of patient co-operation and tumour resistance to anticancer therapy should be carefully evaluated before deciding on further anticancer treatment.

Recommended reading

1. Holland, J. F. and Frei, E. (1982). *Cancer Medicine*. (Philadelphia: Lea and Febiger).
2. De Vita, V. T. Jr., Hellman, S. and Rosenberg, S. (1982). *Cancer Principles and Practice of Oncology*. (Philadelphia, Toronto: J. B. Lippincott).
3. Swerdlow, M. (ed.) (1986). *The Therapy of Pain*. 2nd Edn. (Lancaster: MTP Press).

4. WHO (1985). Essential drugs for cancer therapy. *Bull. WHO*, **63** (6), 998–1002.
5. Price, P., Hoskin, P. J., Easton, D., Austin, D., Palmer, S. G. and Yarnold, J. R. (1986). Prospective randomized trial of single and multifraction radiotherapy schedules in the treatment of painful bony metastases. *Radiother. Oncol.*, **6**, 247–255.

9

Palliative Surgery in Cancer Pain Treatment

A. Azzarelli and S. Crispino

INTRODUCTION

Severe, increasing and resistant pain, if inadequately treated, may be the only or main cause of discomfort in cancer patients. In some clinical situations when radical cure is impossible, appropriate palliative surgical treatment can relieve pain and improve the quality of life or reduce the amount of drugs and other therapies required for the control of pain. The limited life expectancy and the degree of impairment of activity of patients with cancer in advanced stages are frequently important considerations in selecting the appropriate surgical procedure. The aim should be to obtain long lasting relief of pain and other discomforts with the minimum of mutilation and with minimal hospitalization.

GENERAL PRINCIPLES

There are four different types of palliative surgery:

(1) Direct palliative surgery solves contingent and serious clinical situations (e.g. simple mastectomy, colostomy) or improves the therapeutic effect of radio- and chemotherapy so reducing the need for pharmacological control of pain.

(2) Indirect palliative surgery is the ablation of endocrine glands, which is effective with metastatic endocrine-related tumours (e.g. ovariectomy for advanced breast cancer and epididimectomy for prostatic carcinoma).

(3) Mediate palliative surgery which provides a direct access to a tumour-bearing area for radio- or chemotherapy (e.g. intra-arterial infusion chemotherapy).

(4) Surgery of the peripheral nervous system to interrupt transmission of noxious impulses at different CNS levels.

Surgical palliative treatment is often performed in advanced stages of the disease and the risk of mortality and postoperative morbidity may be high.

The use of palliative surgery in association with radiation therapy or chemotherapy can often result in more limited resection, better quality of life, and less need for hazardous surgical treatment.

PALLIATIVE SURGERY METHODS

The more important indications for palliative treatment in cancer patients are shown in Table 8.

ABDOMINAL CANCER

Palliative surgery for abdominal cancer is frequently performed for primary or recurrent lesions of the gastrointestinal (GI) tract, which are responsible for intestinal occlusion or painful involvement of the abdominal wall or retroperitoneal structures.

Palliative procedures are also necessary for acute occlusion of the lower urinary tract and for complications due to advanced ovarian cancer or metastatic involvement from a distant primary lesion (e.g. breast cancer).

Intestinal occlusion

This is a frequent complication in advanced colorectal cancer but it is less frequent in tumours of other parts of the gastrointestinal tract.

Table 8 Major clinical conditions requiring palliative surgery for pain

Clinical condition	Tumour	Type of palliative surgery
Breast tumour	Ulcerating Fungating	Simple mastectomy
Abdominal cancer		
Intestinal occlusion	Colorectal carcinoma ovarian, peritoneal carcinomatosis	Colostomy GI bypass
Intractable pelvic pain	Colorectal carcinomas	Intra-arterial infusion (5FU, Nitrogen mustard)
Serious ascites	Breast, ovarian cancer	Peritoneovenous shunt
Acute urinary tract occlusion	Upper tract: flank and retroperitoneal tumour Pelvic tract: cancer of cervix, prostate, rectum	Nephrostomy Cutaneous ureterostomy Cystostomy
Rectovesical fistula		Colostomy
Rectovaginal fistula		Colostomy
Tumours of the extremities		
Large lesions	Sarcomas, epithelial tumours, metastic visceral tumours	Reductive surgery (amputation) Disarticulation
Pathological fracture	Metastases from lung, breast, prostatic, renal, thyroid carcinomas Primary advanced bone and soft tissue tumours	Amputation Prostheses Pins
Axial nervous system involvement		
Spinal cord compression	Metastases from lung, breast, prostatic, renal, thyroid carcinomas Lymphomas, sarcomas	Decompressive laminectomy

The presence of distant metastases and locally unresectable tumours limits the possibility of radical surgical treatment. In these cases, a GI bypass or colostomy usually solves mechanical problems, and improves the relative quality and length of the patient's remaining life. Obstruction of the small bowel is common in carcinomatosis of the peritoneal cavity (secondary to GI, ovarian or breast cancer). Surgical procedures are rarely helpful for long periods of time, and the surgical approach may be difficult.

After accurate evaluation of possible therapies, an attempt should be made to remove or bypass the intestinal obstruction, if possible. When surgery is not really feasible, a nasogastric tube or parenteral nutrition may restore adequate performance.

Intractable pelvic pain

Intractable pain due to local spread is frequent in patients with advanced pelvic neoplasms (anorectal, urinary bladder, gynaecological cancers and sarcomas). More recently intra-arterial infusion chemotherapy has been investigated for palliative purposes. This procedure is performed by means of a polyethylene catheter percutaneously placed usually in both the internal iliac arteries. It is claimed to have low toxicity, an acceptable morbidity and complication rate, and produces effective pain-relief for about 6–8 weeks, depending on the kind of tumour and its responsivity to the chosen drug. Colorectal cancer has been treated with infusion of 5 FU, urinary bladder cancer and sarcomas with doxorubicin.

Ascites

Conspicuous malignant ascites causes severe discomfort and respiratory impairment. The basic treatment is paracentesis, although it is effective only for a short time and requires repeating. Intracavitary radiocolloidal agents, external beam radiation, and intracavitary chemotherapy have also been used but with poor results.

Peritoneovenous shunt can provide effective palliation of malignant ascites, not controlled by medical treatment, in 70–80% of instances. The technique employs a special Le Veen's silicon strut valve or Denver valve at the peritoneal end of the catheter that prevents blood regurgitation and takes advantage of the pumping action of respiration. The position of the venous end of the tip is controlled by a postoperative X-ray of the chest.

Survival is not modified. The systemic re-infusion in the venous blood of malignant cells eventually viable in the ascites, is not relevant from the clinical point of view. In fact all patients with intractable malignant ascites will die before the appearance of any other metastatic spread.

Shunting is not recommended in patients with hepatic or renal failure, with blood ascitic fluid or with serious coagulation disorders. At the present time if the anticipated survival period is very short (less than 1 month) paracentesis is the treatment of choice; otherwise shunt provides good palliation.

Acute urinary tract occlusion

Acute flank pain may be a clinical feature of sudden obstruction of the urinary tract. In this event the immediate release of obstruction is essential to control pain and to prevent renal impairment, uraemia and infection.

Ureteral obstruction can be due to infiltration by retroperitoneal masses or, in the pelvic tract, from cancer of the cervix, bladder, prostate, ovary or rectum. The majority of upper urinary tract obstructions require urinary diversion by nephrostomy or cutaneous ureterostomy. Obstruction of the lower tract may be palliated by suprapubic cystostomy. These techniques can be performed under local anaesthesia.

TUMOURS OF THE EXTREMITIES OR TRUNK

Large lesions of the extremities

Primary sarcoma, epithelial tumour or metastatic growths in the limbs can be very large and, by infiltration or compression, can cause functional limitation, deformity and pain.

Indications for surgery are: (a) gross dimension, (b) ulceration with bleeding and infection, (c) non-responsiveness to chemo- or radiation therapy, (d) intractable pain, (e) functional limitation, (f) psychological discomfort.

The surgical treatment consists in removal of the lesion, if possible by conservative surgery but if necessary by radical surgery which frequently involves amputation or disarticulation.

Pathological fracture

Pathological fractures induce pain and functional disability. In some cases of relatively slow local progression (e.g. in metastases from breast, thyroid or renal carcinoma) surgical treatment is justified; in fact the insertion of pins or prostheses has a useful functional and analgesic palliative role. The choice between amputation, prosthetic replacement and no therapy, should be determined by the patient's life expectancy, the degree of emergency, the technical difficulties and the estimated length of the hospitalization and rehabilitation period.

(1) Patient life expectancy depends on the kind of tumour and stage. Bone metastases from thyroid or breast cancer can allow years of survival and conservative surgery and prosthetic replacement are therefore indicated. On the other hand, bone metastases from lung oat-cell carcinoma should be treated only with a cast or other external brace; primary large sarcomas are best treated by amputation.

(2) Technical difficulties – the choice of conservative surgery and prosthetic replacement when indicated should be carried out with minimal diagnostic procedures and limited hospitalization. When possible it should be performed in the institute where the primary oncological lesion was treated.

(3) Short rehabilitation time should, for the same reason, follow the conservative surgery.

AXIAL NERVOUS SYSTEM INVOLVEMENT

Spinal cord compression

The most common tumours which can produce spinal cord compression are primary carcinomas, lymphomas, sarcomas and metastatic lung, breast, renal thyroid and prostatic carcinomas.

The surgical treatment of this syndrome consists of decompressive laminectomy preceded by myelography in order to establish the site of the compressive lesion. The surgical procedure should be performed as soon as possible and certainly within 24 hours after the appearance of the first neurological symptom. Complete neurological recovery rarely occurs if the operation is delayed.

In patients with chemo-radiosensitive tumours, such as lymphomas, or where laminectomy is not indicated for any other reason or if the spinal cord compression has slowly increased, the use of radio-chemotherapy can produce effective results (see Chapter 8).

Recommended reading

1. Gennari, L. (1979). Palliative surgery. Advances in pain research and therapy. In Bonica, J. J. and Ventafridda, V. (eds.) *Advances in Pain Research and Therapy.* Vol. 2, pp. 175–83. (New York: Raven Press).
2. Veronesi, U. (1973). Non curative surgery. In: Holland, F. J. and Frei, E. (eds.) *Cancer Medicine.* pp. 530–4. (Philadelphia: Lea and Febiger).

10

Role of Chemical Neurolysis and Local Anaesthetic Infiltration

M. Swerdlow

PAIN RELIEF BY SOMATIC NERVE BLOCK

Introduction

Nerve blocks interrupt nerve function. They can be used to produce a temporary (local anaesthetic) or a long lasting (neurolytic) effect. Temporary blocks can be helpful diagnostically in deciding which nerve or nerves are involved; nerve blocks can also be used to provide lasting analgesia by neurolysis in a specific anatomical area. Nerve blocks are most useful for treatment of patients with localized pain which is severe and persistent, has not responded to the oncological treatment and is inadequately controlled by drug therapy either because of insufficient pain relief or excessive side-effects. For less localized severe pain neurosurgical measures are usually more effective but if such neurosurgery is not available more extensive chemical neurolysis may be carefully applied.

General principles

The following are the general principles which must be adhered to in using nerve blocks in cancer pain management:

(1) Find out the cause of the pain so that the correct block can be applied.

(2) First make sure that the pain syndrome will not respond to primary antitumour therapies such as radiation therapy, chemotherapy or surgery if these are available.

(3) Learn how to apply these nerve blocks, their indications and risks.

(4) Inform the patient of the principles and the potential benefits and risks before carrying out the procedure.

(5) Use radiographic control if it is available: it will make the local anaesthetic and neurolytic placement easier and safer especially in the application of sympathetic blocks. However X-ray control is not necessary for subarachnoid neurolysis.

(6) Deafferentation pain does not respond to somatic nerve blocks.

(7) Use neurolytic block early in the management of patients with pain in the coeliac plexus. Local anaesthetic blocks, repeated if necessary, are indicated early in patients with pain of sympathetic origin.

(8) Nerve blocks are not always adequate alone; they may need to be combined with analgesic drug therapy, neurosurgery and/or physical therapy.

(9) The most common types of pain to be managed with nerve blocks are localized somatic pain involving only two or three dermatomes, visceral pain of coeliac plexus origin or limb pain from involvement of the sympathetic nervous system.

We must stress that nerve blocks will only be necessary in about 20% of patients with cancer pain if analgesic drugs are used properly.

Injection of a neurolytic solution onto the nerves of the pain pathway can often give satisfactory analgesia if the pain is not widespread. Pain in the trunk or limbs due to cancerous involvement of somatic nerves can be relieved most effectively and simply by the injection of the roots of the spinal cord. For head and neck pain and for some cases of very localized trunk pain, due to somatic nerve involvement, neurolysis of peripheral nerves can sometimes be of value. Pain due to involvement of the sympathetic supply to the limbs will often be reduced by sympathetic nerve block.

Spinal neurolysis

The injection of a neurolytic agent to destroy spinal nerve roots is a relatively simple and painless procedure but it may cause functional complications; it can be carried out on patients in poor general condition and the elderly. Spinal root neurolysis does not require special equipment and facilities and it can therefore be made widely available even in small local hospitals. It can be repeated or extended if the first attempt is inadequate. The objective is to deposit the solution as accurately as possible on the target nerve(s); very little neurolytic solution is needed and the risk of involving neighbouring structures should therefore be minimal. The aim should be to destroy only two or three nerve roots at one time. The results of spinal injection are less satisfactory when the pain is widespread or when it is poorly localized. Spinal neurolysis should be used only for somatic pain; it will be relatively ineffective in visceral pain (see p. 122), 'incident pain' (see pp. 114 and 122) or deafferentation pain (see pp. 14 and 86).

It is important to use an aseptic technique and to ensure absolute sterility of equipment when performing any spinal injection. You should also check the sterility and identity of the solution to be injected and make sure that the ampoule is not out-of-date (see Appendix).

Premedication should be avoided if possible because the full co-operation of the patient is necessary during the localization of the neurolytic solution. The results obtained will improve with practice; with increasing skill and experience, the success rate will rise and the incidence of complications will diminish.

If there is pain in more than one place, the area of most severe pain should be tackled first. If there is bilateral pain the two sides should be treated separately at an interval of a day or two, the more severe side first. Removing a severe pain may unmask a less severe pain elsewhere which previously wasn't noticed and this should be relieved by suitable opioid medication or by further nerve block if indicated.

The nerve roots of the spinal cord can be blocked via two routes – *subarachnoid* or *extradural*.

Subarachnoid neurolysis

Intrathecal injection is the easiest and the most useful and effective method of blocking the spinal cord roots. The object of the method is to apply a neurolytic solution to the spinal posterior nerve roots which carry pain impulses from the affected dermatomes. The agents commonly used for subarachnoid neurolysis are phenol and absolute alcohol (for preparation details see Appendix). Phenol (5–7%) is used in solution in glycerine. Alcohol and phenol give similar results in practice: the choice depends to some extent on the experience and training of the administrator. For the beginner, phenol will be found easier to handle.

Lumbar puncture at the dermatome level of the pain (Figure 8) and correct positioning of the patient during injection will help to ensure that the neurolytic agent will move to the roots which need to be

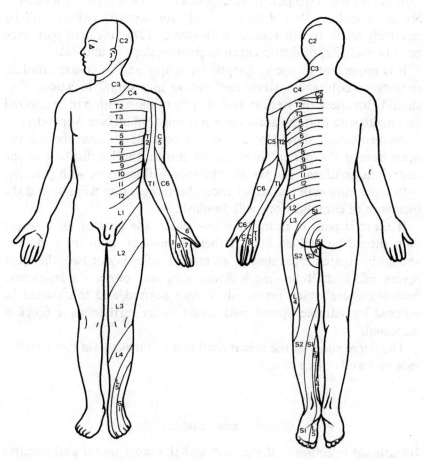

Figure 8 Sensory dermatone chart

destroyed. Subarachnoid neurolysis normally produces analgesia without appreciable sensory loss. It has the further advantage that the block is unlikely to result in more than temporary motor weakness because the posterior spinal roots contain few motor fibres.

Unfortunately the neurolytic agent will produce some destruction of all types of nerve fibres (and other tissues) with which it comes into contact but if the recommended dose and concentration is injected in the right place it is unlikely to cause more than temporary weakness or loss of sensibility. The duration of pain relief and the complications produced appear to be directly related to the amount of nerve fibre destruction. The use of high concentrations and large doses of solution increases the risk of neurological damage and meningeal reaction. Following chemical neurolysis there is a gradual re-generation of nerve fibres so that in time the pain returns but the block can then be repeated to provide a further period of relief.

In general the earlier the patient is referred for treatment the better the chance of achieving good relief as explained on p. 10.

Technique – To perform segmental neurolytic block with phenol at all levels above the lumbosacral region, lie the patient on the painful side on an operating room table (Figure 9). Phenol in glycerine is very hyperbaric (i.e. much heavier than CSF); to introduce it to the posterior nerve roots the patient must be tilted 45° backwards as in Figure 10. A solution of phenol in glycerine is viscid and is difficult to inject through a 20 or 21 gauge spinal needle. The injection will be made easier by using a 1 ml tuberculin-type syringe; this has the added advantage that it prevents any temptation to inject more than 1 ml of

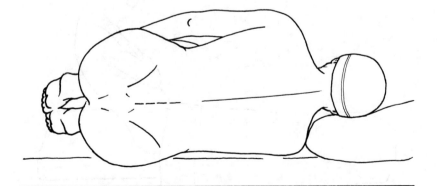

Figure 9   Lateral lumbar puncture position

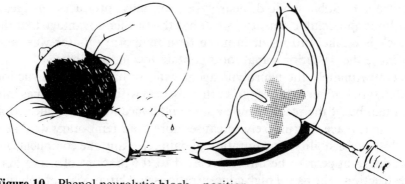

Figure 10   Phenol neurolytic block – position

solution and it facilitates the slow injection of tiny increments of solution. After injection into the CSF the phenol is gradually released from the glycerine; this helps to limit spread of the phenol and achieves a better localization of phenol to the nerve root tissue. When phenol is injected the patient feels warmth or tingling or a prickly feeling in the distribution of nerve roots being affected by the phenol. If on injecting the first 0.2 ml these sensations are more than one dermatome away from the level of pain, it is better to withdraw the spinal needle and re-insert it at the correct level if this can easily be done. (However, if it was very difficult to perform lumbar puncture do not reposition the needle but tilt the table to make the phenol run to the target nerve roots.) A dose of 0.5–1 ml is used for pain at thoracic and cervical levels; at lumbosacral levels the dose should not exceed 0.5 ml.

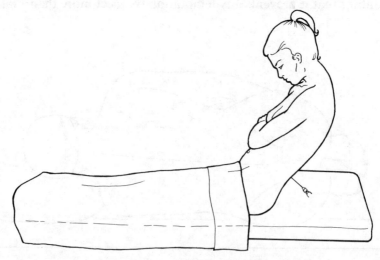

Figure 11   Position for lumbosacral phenol injection

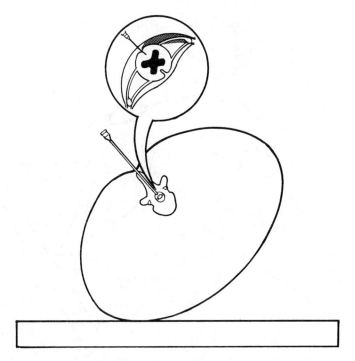

Figure 12   Alcohol neurolytic block – position

Alcohol is very hyperbaric so when it is to be used the patient must be positioned so that the posterior nerve roots to be blocked are situated above the point of entry of the alcohol (Figure 12). When alcohol comes in contact with the spinal nerve roots the patient will feel a painful or burning sensation for a short time. The patient must be warned of this and told to keep still to avoid undue spread of the alcohol in the CSF. The total dose of alcohol should normally not exceed 2 ml and it should be given slowly in small increments using a 2 ml syringe.

Treatment of pain in the *perineal and rectal* area presents difficulties because of the risk of bladder and rectal involvement if the neurolytic agent affects the upper sacral nerve roots. (If incontinence is already present and the patient has an indwelling catheter, this problem does not arise.) When there is pain in the perineum and the buttock or thigh on one side only, a unilateral block will sometimes produce good relief without complications. The patient should be sat up on the operating table or trolley and the spinal needle inserted at L5–S1 interspace. An attempt can be made to get a unilateral block by leaning the patient back to the 45° position and tilting him towards the painful

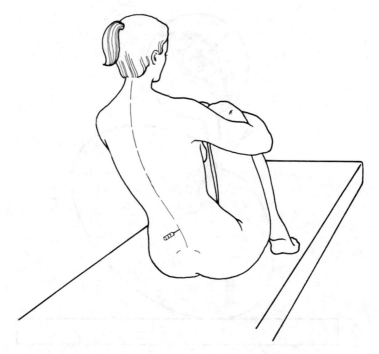

Figure 13   Unilateral lumbosacral block for left side pain

side (Figure 13). The injection of up to 0.5 ml 5% phenol is now given very slowly and the patient maintained in the tilted position for 20 min. In a patient with perineal pain there is frequently marked tenderness on pressure over the perianal area. The disappearance of this tenderness after the block is a good prognostic sign. If the injection is unsuccessful, then a day or two later he should be given a slow intrathecal injection of 0.3–0.5 ml 5% phenol leaning straight back in the midline (Figure 10). An alternative method is caudal block with phenol (see p. 116).

If the pain is in the *mid-thoracic region* (T4–9) arachnoid puncture can be difficult because of the overlapping vertebral spines (Figure 14). If you find it difficult to get the needle to enter the theca at this level, you will find it easier to introduce the spinal needle in an interspace either below (e.g. T10–11) or above (e.g. T2–3) the desired cord level. The table can then be tilted to make the injected neurolytic solution run towards the target section of the spinal cord. A dose of 1–1.5 ml phenol will then be necessary to travel the necessary distance to the desired nerve roots. The results of cervical injections are less satisfactory than those at lower levels of the cord.

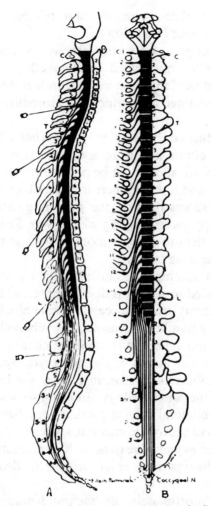

A   B

Figure 14   Spinal column and nerve roots (anatomical)

Alcohol may produce better results than phenol at cervical and upper thoracic levels. The procedure gives best results when the thoracic wall only is involved; with invasion of pleura or lung tissue the relief will be unsatisfactory.

Postinjection management – The patient should be nursed lying flat on his back for the first 24 hours to reduce the risk of postlumbar puncture headache. For the same reasons he should be encouraged to drink as much as possible. A spinal tap can produce a 150 ml CSF loss. It is important to note whether any motor defects develop following the block and whether there is normal bowel and bladder function. If complications arise, then corrective and rehabilitatory treatment should be started at once (see below).

Most patients will get good or moderately good quality relief but 20–30% of patients are not helped by this method. The duration of relief after an intrathecal injection varies considerably but usually 1–3 months relief is obtained after which the procedure can be repeated if necessary.

If the block produces only a day or two of relief, a further injection should be given to obtain a satisfactory result. If this repeat block is ineffective a third block should not be performed because it would be unlikely to succeed and it would increase the risk of complications.

If the block is successful and the pain is greatly relieved it is important to get any joints moving which were formerly painful to move, to get the patient to become more active and try to reduce the amount of analgesic drug taken.

Depression often accompanies chronic pain and the psychological state must be attended to so that it does not prevent the patient from returning to full activity after a successful nerve block (see p. 23).

Failure – There are a number of reasons why subarachnoid neurolysis may fail to give pain relief. Inflammatory changes and cancerous infiltration may prevent access of the neurolytic agent to the nerve roots. Sometimes failure occurs because there is a large sympathetic nervous element in the pain aetiology (for example, visceral abdominal pain, for which a bilateral coeliac plexus block (see p. 122) will be required). Intrathecal neurolytic injections will also fail to relieve pain on movement (*incident pain*) due to pathological fracture of a vertebra or other bone; in these patients relief can be provided by appropriate splinting.

Complications – Unfortunately subarachnoid neurolysis sometimes causes complications. The complications are usually transient but some persist and cause difficulties in patient management. Paraesthesiae and numbness are common; they give little trouble and are usually short-lasting. Less common and much more serious complications are muscular paresis, hypotonia and interference with rectal and vesical sphincter action which is usually temporary. If muscular weakness does occur following neurolysis, physiotherapy (exercises) and the use of a walking aid will help early mobilization (see Chapter 13).

If the patient develops retention of urine or dribbling incontinence, a catheter should be inserted and antibiotic therapy commenced. The catheter should be removed at intervals to test for recovery of micturition.

Epidural neurolysis

The epidural route rather than subarachnoid may be used (1) for neurolytic block of the sacral somatic nerve output in cases where the risk of interference with bowel or bladder function would be particularly serious; (2) for blocks of the cervical nerve outflow; (3) in hospitalized patients by employing an epidural catheter to give repeat doses of local anaesthetic solution, thereby providing a continuous period of pain relief.

The extradural space lies between the spinal dura and the vertebral canal (Figure 15). The space contains a plexus of veins, the spinal arteries, some lymphatics and adipose tissue. The spinal nerve roots pass across the space to reach the intravertebral foramina. If local anaesthetic solution is injected into the extradural space it will block the spinal nerve roots as they cross the space. If a neurolytic solution is injected the pain relief will last longer. However, the administration of a single dose of neurolytic agent by the epidural route for somatic nerve destruction is not usually as effective as intrathecal block. Usually the block produced is less clearly unilateral, is less intense and is of shorter duration than a subarachnoid neurolytic block.

Technique – The patient should lie on his side on the table with the painful side underneath. The back should be swabbed with antiseptic solution. An 8 cm long 18 SWG Tuohy epidural needle or thin-walled

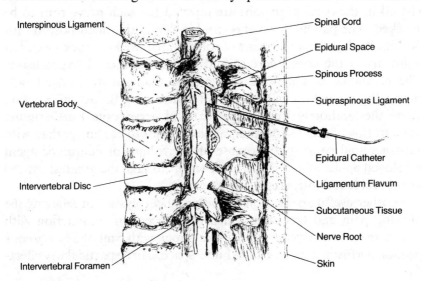

Figure 15   Epidural injection

spinal needle can be used. A wheal is made by injection of 1 ml 1% lignocaine solution into the skin over the middle of the interspinous space where the needle is to be introduced; this should correspond to the spinal root level of the middle of the painful dermatomes (Figure 8). The needle is inserted through the wheal and advanced in the midline through the supraspinous ligament and then through the interspinous tissue until it reaches the dense *ligamentum flavum*. If the needle is now gently pushed through this ligament there will be a sudden loss of resistance which denotes that the tip of the needle is now in the extradural space (Figure 15). (If CSF exudes, the needle has been pushed too far and has pierced the dura.)

Injection of 1 ml of air or dilute local anaesthetic solution will be found to be easy and unresisted. Identification of the epidural space can be made easier by placing a drop of water in the aperture of the hub of the needle; the drop will be sucked in when the needle tip enters the epidural space. If blood exudes when the needle enters the space it is probably better not to proceed with the injection but to try again later.

After the needle has been positioned in the epidural space the patient is tilted backwards into the 45° position as for intrathecal phenol (Figure 10).

A test dose of 3 ml 1% lignocaine is now injected and after ensuring that the solution has not been deposited intrathecally, (e.g. inability to move the feet) 2 ml of a 7–10% solution of phenol in glycerine/water (1.5 ml in the cervical region) are injected for each nerve root to be blocked. The patient is retained on his side in the tilted position for 40 min. With the small volume of solution required to block just a few segments of the cord, there should be little danger of hypotension. The technique is somewhat less precise than subarachnoid block, especially because the patient cannot state during the actual injection where the solution is situated relative to the nerve roots. Furthermore, the duration of relief with epidural block tends to be shorter than with subarachnoid neurolysis. Because of the volume of neurolytic agent employed epidurally, it is most important to take the greatest care to avoid accidental intrathecal injection.

Another useful application of epidural neurolysis is in relieving the burning pain and tenesmus which often occur in conjunction with carcinoma of the rectum. An epidural block with 5 ml of 5% aqueous phenol, performed in the T12–L1 interspace, can be particularly effective.

A special use of the epidural route is by *caudal block*. If phenol is injected into the caudal canal with the table tilted foot-down, it is possible to block the 4th and 5th sacral nerve roots without endangering the upper sacral nerves. In this way it may be possible to relieve perineal pain without causing bladder or rectal complications. (For details of technique see Recommended reading.)

If the patient is hospitalized or mostly confined to bed, valuable use can be made of the epidural route by employing an indwelling epidural catheter (Figure 15). This is a fine catheter made of nylon or polyvinyl chloride which is passed through an 18 SWG needle so that a few centimetres of the catheter lie within the extradural space; the needle is then removed. Such a catheter may safely be left *in situ* for several weeks if a Millipore bacterial filter is attached to the free end of the catheter and care is taken with sterility. Repeat injections can be given into the epidural space via the filter and catheter as often as necessary to maintain a high degree of analgesia. The solution injected may be 2% aqueous phenol in 0·5–1 ml doses or local anaesthetic solution (bupivacaine 0.25%, 2 ml per nerve root).

The plunger should be withdrawn to exclude CSF or blood before injecting the solution into the catheter. Phenol has the advantage that repeat injections are required much less frequently (every 1 or 2 weeks). It is essential that there is adequate surveillance if this catheter form of therapy is used. Neurological sequelae are unusual after epidural neurolytic block.

When nerve roots are inflamed by pressure of infiltrated lymph nodes, relief of pain can be obtained by injecting through the catheter a solution of 80 mg methylprednisolone in 10–20 ml distilled water with 2 ml 1% lignocaine plain.

Peripheral nerve blocks

Chemical neurolysis of peripheral nerves does not usually produce long lasting pain relief in cancer patients. However, occasionally with severe very localized pain a peripheral nerve block may be worthwhile.

If peripheral neurolysis is to be employed, it is important first to carry out a block with local anaesthetic solution to confirm that the correct nerve is being blocked, that the block actually relieves the pain and that any side-effects produced are acceptable. It is unwise to perform blocks, especially deep injections such as coeliac plexus block, on patients who are receiving anticoagulants, because of the danger

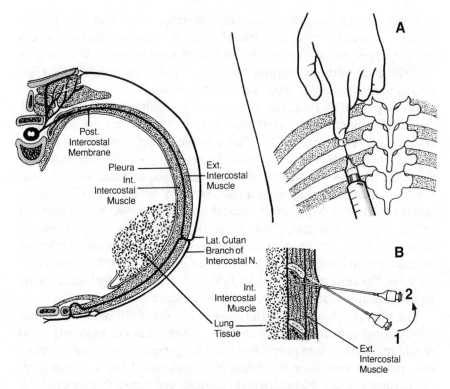

Anatomical sections of the chest wall showing the intercostal nerve.
A. surface view of intercostal nerve injection.
B. Sagittal section at approximately midaxillary line.

Figure 16   Intercostal nerve block

of massive haemorrhage from the muscle tissues through which the needle passes.

Chemical neurolysis of peripheral nerves is best produced with phenol. Injection of neurolytic agents at superficial sites (e.g. intercostal nerve block) can result in skin ulceration. A little air or saline should therefore be injected as the needle is being withdrawn so as not to leave behind a track of neurolytic agent.

Pain due to involvement of one or two intercostal nerves only (e.g. in carcinoma breast or bronchus) can be relieved by *intercostal block* provided that there is no pleural involvement. Usually because of overlap of the nerve supply the two adjacent nerves need to be blocked to obtain a satisfactory result (e.g. pain at L7 level might need block of T6 and 8 as well as T7 intercostal nerve). If the test block is satisfactory it should be repeated using 0.5–1 ml 7% aqueous phenol per intercostal nerve near the angle of rib taking care to avoid puncturing the pleura which would cause pneumothorax (Figure 16). The duration of relief is rarely longer than 2 or 3 weeks.

If there is a rib metastasis with severe pain and localized tenderness at the site of the secondary, the intercostal nerve proximal to the metastasis should be anaesthetized with local anaesthetic solution (e.g. 0.25% bupivacaine). 2 ml (80 mg) of methylprednisolone should then be injected around the tender point in the rib. This often gives several weeks of pain relief. Similarly an injection of bupivacaine and methylprednisolone given into the vicinity of a superficially located bone secondary (e.g. in the scapula), is a simple measure which will often provide a period of pain relief and can be repeated as often as necessary.

Neck, head and facial pain

Pain in the head and neck often presents many problems. There are a number of nerves in the region (i.e. cervical, trigeminal, glossopharyngeal, vagus, superior laryngeal) and block of any one or two of them may prove inadequate to resolve the pain. Spread of the tumour can soon render a satisfactory block ineffective. Also glandular infiltration in the neck region may make needle access impossible.

When neck and facial pain become troublesome and opioid medication is proving inadequate a neurosurgeon and an oncologist should be consulted, if possible, regarding the best means of obtaining relief. If the patient is unsuitable or unfit for such treatment or these therapies are not available, relief by neurolytic block should be considered. Sometimes cervical neurolysis via the epidural route is helpful for neck and shoulder pain.

It is important to apply nerve blockade before the disease is so far advanced that it would be very difficult to carry out any effective nerve blocking procedure. For pain in the head or face, alcohol block of the trigeminal (gasserian) ganglion is performed; absolute alcohol is injected in 0.1 or 0.2 ml increments up to a total of not more than 1 ml. For pain localized to the distribution of a major branch of the trigeminal (i.e. mandibular or maxillary) a dose of 0.5–1 ml alcohol is employed. A preliminary injection of 1 ml 1% lignocaine will confirm that the needle tip is close to the nerve and will also reduce the amount of pain that the patient feels when the alcohol is injected. (For details of these blocks, the reader is referred to Recommended reading.) These procedures require expertise and it is helpful if X-ray control is available; the patient should be referred to the nearest major hospital (see Chapter 13).

Malignant invasion of the *brachial plexus* in carcinoma bronchus and carcinoma breast gives slowly progressive flaccid paresis of the arm with sensory loss commencing distally. Muscle wasting may be hidden by swelling of the arm due to venous and lymphatic obstruction. The pain of brachial plexus involvement can be quite devastating, and if all else fails, including anticonvulsants and antidepressants, chemical neurolysis of the plexus must be considered. For this procedure up to 15 ml absolute alcohol or 1–3% aqueous phenol may be used. Both agents cause considerable pain on injection and for some time afterwards and the patient should be given adequate analgesic medication. Alternatively, a fine catheter can be placed supraclavicularly in the brachial plexus and injections of 10 ml 0.5% bupivacaine given through it as often as necessary for temporary relief.

If the arm is non-functional, 10 ml of absolute alcohol can be injected through the catheter to provide a longer duration of relief. (For technique see Recommended reading.)

Pain from cancer in the region of the apex of the thorax including Pancoast tumour can be most difficult to relieve; it may have a sympathetic element (see below) as well as a somatic one. Many of these patients exhibit motor weakness, neuralgia, trophic changes and burning pain often associated with dysaesthesia or hyperpathia. In addition there may be massive oedema of the arm. Intrathecal or extradural injection of a single dose of neurolytic agent may help to relieve the somatic element of the pain for at least a while. However, a single neurolytic block often fails to produce an adequate duration of relief. Relief of severe pain may sometimes be provided by intermittent administration of 2% phenol solution via an indwelling extradural catheter. Alternatively, extradural local anaesthetic solution may be injected when necessary through an indwelling catheter with millipore filter if adequate supervision is available. Stellate ganglion block (see p. 125) will probably also be necessary.

Myofascial pain

Chronic myofascial pain may occur in patients with cancer. This condition is typified by the presence of 'trigger points' in muscles in the painful region (Figure 17). Trigger points are small tender nodes or even palpable nodules, pressure on which causes sharp pain which

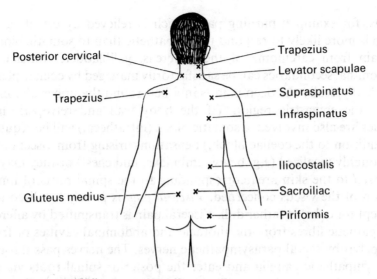

Posterior cervical

Trapezius

Trapezius

Levator scapulae

Supraspinatus

Infraspinatus

Iliocostalis

Gluteus medius

Sacroiliac

Piriformis

Figure 17 Common trigger points

may radiate to other areas, sometimes quite distant. Treatment consists of injection into the trigger point(s) of local anaesthetic solution (e.g. 2–3 ml 0.25% bupivacaine) to break the vicious circle of pain→spasm→pain. The injection will need to be repeated at intervals.

Another simple local anaesthetic injection which can be helpful is for *sacroiliac pain*. Pain and marked tenderness over one or both sacroiliac joints are quite common in middle-aged and older people. They are particularly common in those who have lost a lot of weight and hence in cancer patients. The sacroiliac joint lies just medial to the posterior iliac crest at the lateral margin of the upper sacrum. The fascia covering the joint can usually be reached quite easily with a 4 cm long 22 gauge needle. A dose of 5 ml 0.5% bupivacaine should be injected around the tender area at this site; if effective, the injection will need repeating at intervals.

PAIN RELIEF BY AUTONOMIC NERVE BLOCK

There are many instances where some or all of the pain is due to involvement of autonomic nerves and for which block of this part of the nervous system will be required to obtain pain relief. Careful history and examintion are necessary to elucidate the exact distribution and quality of the pain and its aggravating features. The patient should be examined for signs of abnormal autonomic function (see p.132).

Thus, for example, burning pain which is relieved by elevating the limb is more likely to respond to sympathetic than to somatic block.

Pain from carcinoma of the pancreas, gallbladder, stomach or abdominal secondaries can be satisfactorily managed by coeliac plexus block. Typically the deep pain is in a belt round the upper abdomen from the epigastric region. (If the body wall and retroperitoneal tissues are also involved, a somatic block (intrathecal) will be required in addition to the coeliac block.) Sensations arising from viscera may be roughly localized (e.g. below umbilicus, mid chest) or they may be *referred* to the skin area corresponding to the spinal roots of innervation of the viscus concerned. *Visceral pain* is poorly localized and (except for colic) is rather dull. Visceral pain is transmitted by afferent sympathetic fibres from the thoracic and abdominal cavities or from the pelvis by sacral parasympathetic nerves. The nerves pass through the sympathetic ganglia and enter the posterior spinal roots via the white rami communicantes. Their cell bodies are in the posterior root ganglion.

Coeliac plexus block – technique

The coeliac plexus is situated on the front and both anterolateral aspects of the body of L1 vertebra and the lower half of T12 (Figure 18).

To achieve total blockade of the plexus, bilateral injection is necessary. (The use of an image intensifier (X-ray control) if available will greatly facilitate the correct placement of the needle and preliminary injection of 0.5 ml Conray 280 will confirm that the injected solution is retroperitoneal.)

The patient should be positioned lying prone with a pillow under the abdomen. A line between the posterior iliac crests passes through the space between the 4th and 5th lumbar spines. Count upwards from L4 spine to L1 spine. Make skin wheals with local anaesthetic four fingers breadth to the right and left of the midline and at the level of L1 spine; the wheals must be below (i.e. caudal to) the 12th ribs. Now insert a 16 cm long, 20 gauge needle through the wheal at 45° (Figure 19) to the plane of the back and advance the needle gently with the bevel facing inward and in a slightly cephelad direction. When the point of the needle strikes the body of L1 the needle should be partially withdrawn and re-inserted so that it glances off the anterolateral aspect of the body of the vertebra. The needle is advanced 1 cm past this

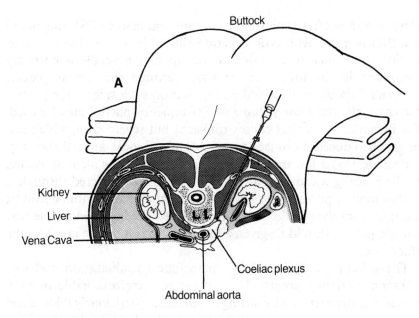

Figure 18   Coeliac plexus (cross-section: anatomical)

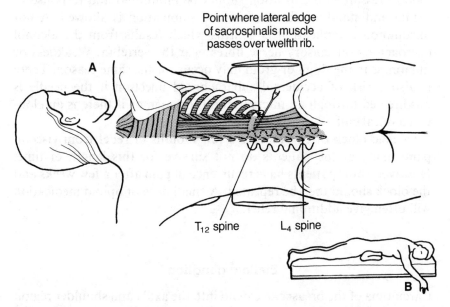

Figure 19   Coeliac plexus block

point and then after aspirating to ensure that neither CSF nor blood is withdrawn the neurolytic injection should be made. There should be little resistance to injection if the tip of the needle is correctly positioned in the loose areolar tissue around the coeliac plexus. 15–20 ml 75% alcohol should be injected on each side of the plexus. Alternatively, the same volume of 7% aqueous phenol may be used. The injection of alcohol causes transient but severe pain, which can be much reduced by injection of 2–3 ml of local anaesthetic (e.g. lignocaine 1%) a few minutes before introducing the alcohol. As the needle is being withdrawn air or saline should be injected through it so that lumbar plexus nerves do not get contaminated with neurolytic solution from the needle. Having completed the injection on the first side the patient should be given a few minutes rest before injecting the other side.

The injection is followed by splanchnic vasodilatation and loss of vasoconstricting ability. The patient is, therefore, liable to have orthostatic hypotension on sitting or standing, particularly if his blood volume is reduced or he is dehydrated. At the completion of the injection each leg should be tightly bound from foot to groin with elastocrepe bandage. If necessary an intravenous infusion should be started and a pressor drug (e.g. ephedrine) given. The circulatory instability can persist for a day or two and for this reason the pulse, blood pressure and hydration should be monitored and response to sitting and standing observed before ambulation is allowed. A not uncommon complication is neuritis which results from the alcohol encroaching on sensory nerve fibres near the vertebra. Weakness or numbness in the thigh or groin may occur for the same reason. There is also a risk of accidental subarachnoid injection if the needle is misdirected through an intervertebral foramen or if there is an elongated dural cuff.

Coeliac block often provides a few months of relief from visceral pain; many of the patients do not survive for this length of time. However, some patients have recurrence of pain after a few weeks and the block should then be repeated. A small dose of opioid medication will often give additional relief.

Stellate ganglion

Carcinoma of the breast can extend into the axilla and shoulder region and cause diffuse burning pain. Following radical mastectomy some patients develop severe burning pain in the scar and in the ipsilateral arm. In the upper thorax also primary and secondary spread sometimes involves sympathetic nerve fibres (either paravertebrally, in the brachial plexus or in the major arm vessels) causing oedema, cyanosis and burning pain in the arm. These are symptoms of sympathetic nerve involvement and in such cases stellate ganglion block will be found valuable.

Technique

The stellate ganglion lies in front of the base of the transverse process of the 7th cervical vertebra (Figure 20). Close to the stellate ganglion are a number of important structures, so that when blocking the ganglion great care must be taken to avoid pneumothorax, intravascular injection, subarachnoid injection or block of the recurrent laryngeal, phrenic or vagus nerves. The ganglion is best approached by an anterior paratracheal route. Lie the patient supine on the table with a small pillow under his neck to extend the head. Insert your

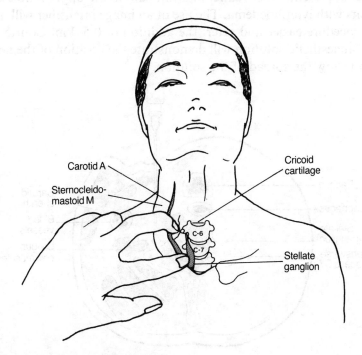

Figure 20   Stellate ganglion block

left index and middle fingers between the sternomastoid muscle and the trachea on the side to be blocked. On deep palpatation at the level of the thyroid cartilage a transverse process will easily be felt – this is usually at C6. Make a skin wheal with 1% lignocaine solution about 1 cm caudal to this palpated transverse process. Insert a 5–7 cm long, 20 gauge needle through the local anaesthetic skin wheal and advance it to contact the transverse process of the 7th cervical vertebra (Figure 21). Now withdraw the needle a millimetre or two and aspirate to make sure that neither blood nor CSF issues from the needle. 5–10 ml of 0.5% lignocaine solution or 0.25% bupivacaine should now be injected with the needle in close proximity to the transverse process. The rapid development of Horner's syndrome (myosis, enophthalamus, ptosis) following injection confirms a successful block. Other signs of a successful block are flushing of the conjunctiva and sclera, flushing of cheek, face, and neck, filling of arm veins and increased arm temperature.

If local anaesthetic block of the stellate ganglion provides appreciable relief it can be repeated each time the block starts to wear off. A series of stellate ganglion blocks with local anaesthetic will often prove helpful in patients with deafferentation pain in the upper limb and in patients with lymphoedema. The use of an image intensifier will make this procedure easier and safer; the addition of 0.5–1 ml Conray 280 to the anaesthetic solution will demonstrate the position of the needle tip and show the spread of the solution.

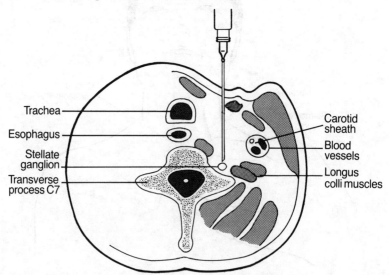

Figure 21   Stellate ganglion (cross-section: anatomical)

Lumbar sympathetic block

Some patients with malignancy in the pelvic region develop burning pain and lymphoedema of the leg. This will probably be relieved by block of the lumbar sympathetic chain. The sympathetic chain lies on the anterolateral aspect of the lumbar vertebrae.

Technique

Lie the patient on his side on a trolley or table with the side to be blocked upwards and the hips flexed. Swab the skin of the back with antiseptic solution and apply sterile towels. Now identify the spine of the 3rd lumbar vertebra. (A line joining the iliac crests passes through the 4th spine or the space between L4 and L5 spines.) Make a skin wheal with local anaesthetic at the level of the L3 spine, four fingers breadth lateral to the midline on the side to be blocked. Through this wheal introduce a 16–20 cm long, 19 gauge needle and advance it in the direction of the body of L3 vertebra, the bevel of the needle facing medially (Figure 22). When the needle strikes the body of the vertebra, it should be withdrawn slightly and the angle of the needle adjusted so that it glides off the anterolateral aspect of the vertebra. After aspirating to make sure that neither blood nor CSF are present in the

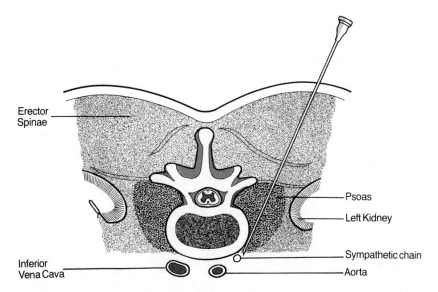

Figure 22   Lumbar sympathetic block

needle, inject 10–15 ml of either 0.5% lignocaine or 0.25% bupivacaine. If this local anaesthetic block produces a marked improvement it should be repeated as often as necessary; if this is not possible consideration should be given to repeating the block with 5 ml of a neurolytic solution a few days later. Sympathetic block with 5–7% phenol should give good results for up to 6 months. A temporary fall of blood pressure may occur especially in elderly and dehydrated patients in which case the patient should be tilted head down and an intravenous infusion started.

Recommended reading

1. Swerdlow, M. (1983). *Relief of Intractable Pain*. 3rd Edn., (Amsterdam: Elsevier Press) p. 147.
2. Moore, D. C. (1986). *Regional Block*. 6th Edn. (Springfield, Ill.: Thomas).
3. Cousins, M. and Bridenbaugh, P. (1980). *Neural Blockade*. (Philadelphia: Lippincott).

11

Practical Neurosurgical Techniques

E. R. Hitchcock

Although many analgesic surgical procedures are beyond the experience or expertise of the general surgeon, a number of techniques are at his disposal, provided he is able to perform a laminectomy and is willing to study the anatomy of the base of the skull.

Nevertheless the procedures to be described are best performed with the facilities of a neurosurgical department available, for even the simplest percutaneous procedure has a risk, admittedly small, of producing an acute condition which may require immediate neurosurgical exploration. However, if neurosurgical expertise is not available the suffering cancer patient should not be denied help which can be given by simple surgery. The practical aspects of analgesic surgery have been emphasized and the procedures are described on an anatomical basis, a general description of the procedure and a description of the technique. More complex procedures are only briefly described although the indications should be understood so that intelligent referral can be made.

GENERAL CONSIDERATIONS

Although we can expect a high rate of pain cure in patients with malignancy we should always choose the procedure which is most

129

likely to give a long duration of pain relief. In making such choices we must be guided by three principles:

The three principles of analgesic surgery

  (i)   Procedures should not add to the patient's disabilities.
 (ii) Relief should be complete and long lasting.
(iii) Analgesia should anticipate areas of pain extension.

(i) Procedures should not add to the patient's incapacity

Many patients with pain due to cancer are already disabled to some extent. Sometimes these incapacities make the choice of procedure easier but sometimes more difficult. For example a patient who has had a rectal resection and uses a urinary catheter can be treated for rectal pain by methods which produce urinary and rectal incontinence; on the other hand a patient with already diminished respiratory function from a pulmonary neoplasm may not tolerate general anaesthesia or lesions which may injure the nervous or mechanical components of respiration.

(ii) Relief should be complete and long lasting

To the patient with malignant pain any residual pain is a constant reminder of his condition.

Before embarking on surgery, therefore, a surgeon should make sure that properly administered analgesic therapy has proved inadequate and he should try to evaluate the contribution of the patient's emotional state to the pain or, conversely, the contribution of pain to the emotional state. Because of these complex inter-relationships many such patients require treatment for both conditions; treating one without the other is doomed to failure. An attempt should also be made to determine whether the pain is visceral, somatic or both. Sympathetic block always fails to relieve pain with a somatic component. An example is pancreatic cancer where, when the disease is confined to the gland, coeliac plexus block is successful but when the disease has extended paravertebrally then somatic pain occurs and interruption of the somatic pain pathway will be needed as well to achieve relief.

The patient's life expectancy has a considerable influence on choice of technique since a short life expectancy permits the use of simple procedures with relatively high recurrence rates.

(iii) Analgesia should anticipate pain extension

Increasing experience with management of patients with pain due to malignancy shows that many conditions begin with fairly localized pain which extends to other areas as the disease advances. An example is oro-mandibular cancer which, although at first localized to one trigeminal division, ultimately involves the adjacent maxillary division and glossopharyngeal and vagal sensory areas. Cancer of the posterior part of the tongue will tend to involve the mandibular division of the lingual nerve, the glossopharyngeal and vagal nerves and, by extension into the cervical lymph glands, the nerves of the cervical plexus.

The pain of metastatic disease is particularly difficult to deal with because so often the site of the next metastasis and resultant pain cannot be calculated. Opioid analgesia may be effective but more general approaches, such as central stereotactic lesions, deep brain stimulation or hypophysectomy should be considered.

Finally, if analgesic surgery is to be done it is best done early. The longer the pain has been present the less chance of successful analgesic surgery.

In the procedures discussed in the following pages, peripheral neurectomy, rhizotomy and cordotomy should be within the competence of any general surgeon.

However, it is the responsibility of all doctors who attend patients with cancer to be aware of all the possible treatments and to be able to recommend, or counsel against, the more specialized procedures.

The aetiology of cancer pain

A common cause of pain is either direct invasion of bone or more commonly metastasis to bone. In the case of vertebral or extradural metastasis the nerves are often compressed and a common story is back pain or girdle pain followed by progressive paraparesis.

With bony tumours of the extremities the surgeon should consider a palliative debulking of the tumour if pain is caused by pressure or even consider amputation. For abdominal pain caused by viscous obstruction such as obstructive jaundice or intestinal obstruction the surgeon will naturally perform some type of by-pass or decompressive procedure (see Chapter 9).

To the surgeon more familiar with the abdomen than the brain and no experience of or access to facilities for hypophysectomy, pain due to hormone-dependent tumours such as prostate or breast can often be effectively relieved by orchidectomy, oophorectomy or adrenalectomy by standard general surgical procedures. Pain may also be due to infection associated with ulceration or obstruction and a course of antibiotics may produce striking relief.

Careful psychological preparation is of great importance and a simple explanation of the procedure (with a muted warning that some readily treatable or brief post-operative pain is inevitable) is worthwhile in the very early stages of operative cancer treatment. Careful siting of incisions to avoid nerve injury and meticulous aseptic technique with gentle tissue handling are all important to reduce the risk of iatrogenic pain.

We are now aware that many patients with pain associated with neoplastic invasion of nerves suffer from the effects of reduction in nerve impulses rather than an increase, the 'deafferentiation syndrome'. This can often only be relieved by stimulation of the proximal nerve pathways.

PROCEDURES

Sympathectomy

Although sensory fibres run within the sympathetic trunks they do not relay there but pass to the dorsal root ganglion and enter the cord in the same way as other afferent fibres. Thus, posterior rhizotomy produces a sympathetic effect within the dermatome. The sympathetic network is large and complex and many fibres by-pass adjacent ganglia so that the effect of sympathectomy may be transient.

Carcinomatous causalgia (reflex sympathetic dystrophy)

This not uncommon condition is caused by invasion of nerves and especially by the invasion of the lumbar or brachial plexuses. The pain is usually a dull burning sensation and the limb is protected against contact with objects, even clothing, because of hyperpathia, an extreme hypersensitivity to sensory stimulation, even light touch, which is interpreted as painful. The limb may be swollen and vasodilated or vasoconstricted with cyanosis and sweating disorders. Less frequently these symptoms occur in the face, head and neck.

Diagnostic sympathetic blocks of the appropriate ganglia (see Chapter 10) are helpful in determining whether sympathectomy will be helpful but there is little, if any, indication for operative sympathectomy in these cases. Relief can be achieved for a longer duration by rhizotomy, although with the disadvantage that usually more than three rhizotomies are required compared to the excision of a single ganglion such as the stellate. One of the major contraindications to sympathetic block or sympathectomy is that the needle or scalpel must traverse tissue infiltrated with neoplasm. There is little, if any, indication for sympathectomy in the treatment of carcinomatous causalgia other than as a procedure in terminal patients.

Peripheral neurectomy

General: The major peripheral nerves are mixed nerves conveying both motor and sensory impulses and very few are purely sensory other than the most distal portions supplying only the skin. Few patients have cancer pain due to lesions limited to skin and superficial neurectomies are unlikely to be successful. The effect of neurectomy is a sensory loss in the areas supplied by the nerve which will include skin and soft tissues and an accompanying paralysis of the muscles supplied by that nerve. Unfortunately, the sensory overlap is large and it is rarely possible to produce adequate analgesia unless a large trunk such as the sciatic nerve is destroyed with a resulting severe and extensive paralysis.

The need to anticipate neoplastic extension implies multiple neurectomies to produce a sufficiently wide area of denervation. Frequently the nerves innervating the painful area are involved by neoplasm and additionally the loss of all sensory impulses may produce dysaesthesia (the 'deafferentiation' syndrome). There is, therefore, little place for neurectomy in the treatment of cancer pain apart from some patients with advanced head and neck cancers or with head pain due to scalp or skull primary or secondary neoplasms. The nerve may be destroyed by an open procedure, which has the merit of precision and certainty of interruption or by percutaneous procedures.

Cranial

Supra-orbital and supra-trochlear neurectomy

Percutaneous: The supraorbital notch is palpated and a 21G (0.4 mm) needle inserted into the foramen. If this cannot be found the injection should be made close to the bone. Approximately 1 ml of absolute alcohol is required (Figure 23).

Open procedure: This is much easier and more effective than an alcoholic injection. Under general anaesthesia a small incision is made in the upper part of the upper eyelid on to the superior orbital rim. The nerve is found passing over the rim and is grasped in a pair of haemostats and pulled out of the foramen. The supra-trochlear branches lie more laterally but can be seen through the same exposure.

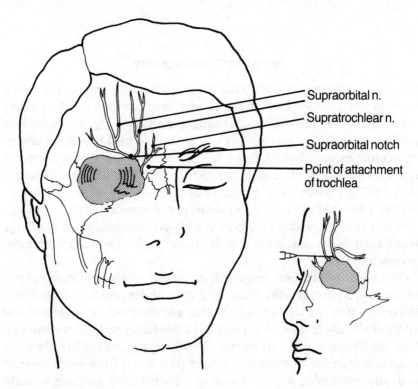

Supraorbital n.

Supratrochlear n.

Supraorbital notch

Point of attachment of trochlea

Figure 23 Supraorbital nerve

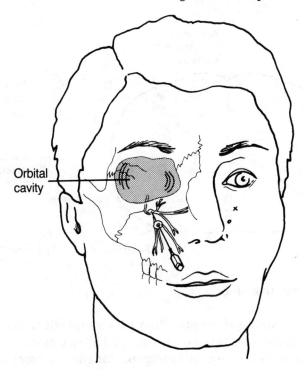

Orbital
cavity

Figure 24 Infraorbital nerve

Infra-orbital neurectomy

Percutaneous: The infra-orbital foramen is palpated with the fore-finger, with the operator standing on the opposite side to the selected nerve. A 21G (0.4 mm) lumbar puncture needle is introduced into the foramen into which a 1 ml injection of absolute alcohol is made (Figure 24). Alternatively an insulated spinal needle may be used with a 5 mm bared tip and a radiofrequency lesion made if the equipment is available.

Open: An incision is made in the gingivo-labial margin and the cheek retracted up and out to expose the nerve entering the foramen. It is grasped in a pair of haemostats and avulsed. The mucosal incision need not be sutured for it heals within a few days during which time the patient should use frequent mouth washes.

Posterior rhizotomy

The fibres conveying pain, temperature and vibration and light touch and proprioceptive sensation diverge from the motor fibres and enter

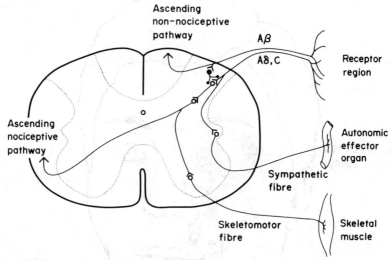

Figure 25 Posterior root fibres

the cord at the posterior roots together with visceral afferents (Figure 25). Section of these roots produces a loss of all these sensations within the areas supplied by the root, including the skin (dermatome), muscle (myotome) and bone (sclerotome). Visceral sensation is also lost but because of the diffuse nature of visceral innervation it is usually only the superficial (angiotomes) that are at all well demarcated.

The effect of posterior rhizotomy is like that of neurectomy, total anaesthesia, but without paralysis. Motor changes can be demonstrated, however, since the loss of the afferent limb of the reflex arc produces hypo- or areflexia and a loss of proprioception results in clumsiness of the affected extremities. In the case of the lumbar nerves this produces transient unsteadiness in walking and, after cervical rhizotomies, transient impairment of fine movements of the hand.

As with neurectomy the loss of sensation may be followed by dysaesthesia which occasionally can be as troublesome as the original pains. Despite adequate rhizotomy, pain may recur after a few months. The reason may be failure to section sufficient roots to denervate an extending neoplasm which now gives pain at the limit of the analgesic zone. Sometimes the pain has the characteristic dysaesthetic character of deafferentation with an aching or burning sensation within the anaesthetized zone.

Rhizotomy is an excellent operation for most patients with cancer pain, especially those with a prognosis of less than six months. The major objection to rhizotomy for cancer pain is that because of the

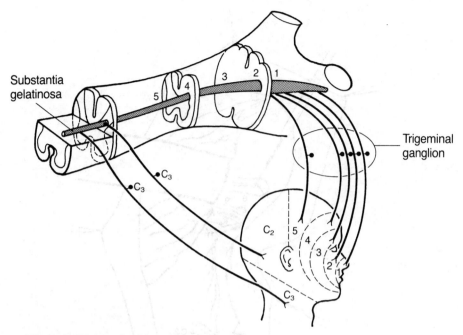

Figure 26 Trigeminal ganglion

extensive sensory overlap it is necessary to section at least two roots above and two roots below as well as the affected root. In the extremities this is a lesser objection because overlap is less and it is often possible to limit the section to two or three roots. Apart from the contiguous areas there is also little overlap between the trigeminal and the cranial nerves and between the trigeminal nerve and the second cervical invasion. Cranial rhizotomy, therefore, tends to be a lesser procedure than elsewhere and more successful in dealing with cancer pain of the head (Figure 26).

Trigeminal rhizotomy produces extensive deep anaesthesia over the face and mouth. The open method has been supplanted by the simpler and safer percutaneous radiofrequency rhizotomy. The surgeon must remember the advancing nature of oro-facial neoplasms and anticipate future areas of pain, seeking to prevent this by choosing more extensive procedures if these are available. Extension of neoplasia, especially cervical invasion, is likely and a posterior fossa exposure enables the upper cervical roots of C2, 3 and 4 to be sectioned together with the lower cranial nerves (Figure 27).

Posterior rhizotomy is most useful in dealing with upper body pain such as that due to lung or breast cancer. An extensive denervation may be required of as many as eight roots from midcervical to upper

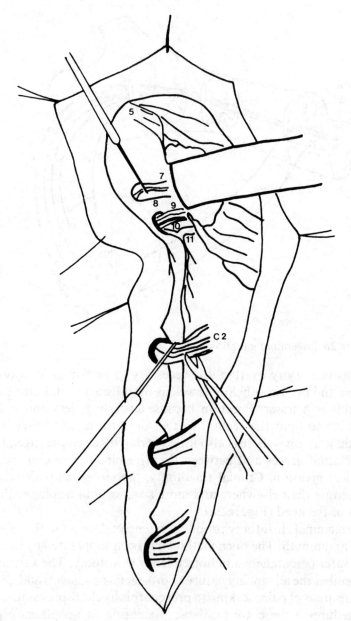

Figure 27 Exposure of cervical roots

thoracic and a corresponding extensive laminectomy or multiple percutaneous rhizotomies.

There are fewer indications for thoracic rhizotomy except for well-
localized tumours such as those invading the lower chest wall, when

a relatively limited rhizotomy may be successful. The relief of pain over more than four truncal dermatomes by open rhizotomy makes it a fearsome procedure, since a very extensive laminectomy is required and such patients are often in poor condition.

An alternative procedure is cordotomy but if this is impossible for any reason then percutaneous rhizotomy should be considered. The root may be destroyed by the injection of neurolytic substances or preferably by radiofrequency heating. The latter technique has the advantage of allowing adjustment of needle and electrode based on radiological demonstration of the electrode tip and from observation of the effects of electrical stimulation. Cryo-destruction of the root (see Recommended Reading) confers no benefits over radiofrequency and is less effective and convenient.

Sacral rhizotomy is a comparatively minor operation which seeks to produce anaesthesia over the involved dermatomes without causing bladder disorder. This implies section below S2 or preserving at least one S2 root. It is indicated for patients with perineal pain due to rectal or prostatic cancer but the anaesthesia produced is often very limited. Both posterior and anterior roots are severed by a single procedure exposing the dura at the lumbo-sacral interspace and sectioning the whole dural sleeve between ligatures. Although by section below the S2 root bladder function may be preserved, the method is best reserved for those whose bladder is already paralysed.

Posterior rhizotomy

Cranial

Trigeminal rhizotomy

Percutaneous: The patient is pre-medicated and an intravenous anaesthetic such as methohexitone or thiopentone is given. The patient lies supine with the head slightly extended. The 20 gauge needle should have a short bevel and be insulated up to 0.5 to 1 centimetre from the tip. It is inserted one inch from the angle of the mouth of the zygoma heading for the foramen ovale (Figure 28). An image intensifier is useful for those inexperienced with the technique. The needle is advanced until the foramen is penetrated and the position is checked by a lateral X-ray and a submentovertical view. The point of the needle should not advance past the clivus. On withdrawal of the stilet there is usually a loss of CSF, or this can be obtained by aspiration.

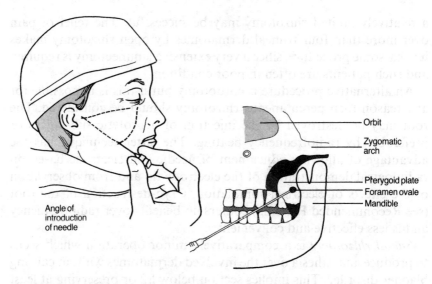

Orbit

Zygomatic arch

Pterygoid plate
Foramen ovale
Mandible

Angle of
introduction
of needle

Figure 28 Gasserian ganglion block

If a radiofrequency generator is available this is preferable to neuro-lytic injection. The temperature monitoring electrode is then inserted through the needle and a radiofrequency lesion made. An earth lead is used either by a flat plate electrode on the shoulder or by a needle electrode inserted into the temporalis muscle.

Electrical stimulation is made at low frequency, 2 Hz, which usually produces temporalis and masseter contraction. The patient is then allowed to awaken and stimulation at 50 Hz made. This produces facial paraesthesia and pain in one or more trigeminal divisions. In contrast to the use of this technique for trigeminal neuralgia, for the relief of cancer pain an attempt should be made to produce deep analgesia which can be confirmed by allowing the patient to awaken and testing for loss of sensation by pinprick.

A radiofrequency lesion is made at 65°C for 60 seconds and repeated incrementally to 70°C and then 75°C stages until analgesia or anaes-thesia is produced.

Alcoholic or phenolic rhizotomy

This is a much simpler procedure than radiofrequency rhizotomy and requires the minimum of apparatus. It is, however, less controllable. The procedure is similar to radiofrequency rhizotomy in the first stages but can usually be performed under local anaesthesia. A tuberculin syringe containing 0.5 ml of absolute alcohol is attached to the needle after insertion and portions of 0.1 ml solution injected, stopping to check sensation after each injection. Alternatively 5% phenol in glycerine can be used but in this case, since the solution is hyperbaric, the patient should be sitting up with the head flexed so that the needle points upwards after insertion.

For both procedures the risk is that the solution will diffuse into the posterior fossa and destroy cranial nerves. Careful technique and incremental injections reduce this risk, although the risk of corneal anaesthesia is very high. In patients with terminal disease these hazards are often acceptable.

Radiofrequency glossopharyngeal rhizotomy

Although trigeminal rhizotomy relieves facial pain and pain in the anterior two-thirds of the tongue, the glossopharyngeal and vagal nerves innervate the posterior third of tongue, the oropharynx, epipharynx and larynx together with part of the auditory meatus. Glossopharyngeal rhizotomy is particularly useful for neoplasms which produce pain on speaking or swallowing. In pain due to oropharyngeal neoplasms, pain is often experienced in both trigeminal and glossopharyngeal territories so that both rhizotomies are required.

The nerve may be destroyed by radiofrequency current or alcohol or phenol solutions and differs from trigeminal rhizotomy only in the angles of needle insertion. The entry point is one inch (2.5 cm) from the labial commissure and the needle is directed more posteriorly than for penetration of the foramen ovale. The needle point is directed to the tragus or on a plane 40° inferior to a line passing through the inferior orbital margin and internal auditory meatus. This is approximately 15° more posterior than the angle used to enter the foramen ovale. The needle then enters the jugular foramen and both glossopharyngeal and vagal nerves can be stimulated. It is also directed approximately 10° lateral to a plane passing through the pupil. The position is checked by lateral and submentovertical X-rays. Electrical stimulation should produce symptoms referrable to the ninth and tenth nerves. Stimulation at less than 0.5 volt produces sensations in the tonsillar fossa, the pharynx and internal auditory meatus. Care should be taken to monitor heart rate as bradycardia may be produced and should be avoided by small adjustments in needle position. This is not as simple a procedure as trigeminal rhizotomy and practice with a cadaver or at least a skull base is strongly recommended.

Spinal

Percutaneous

Cervical: It is helpful to fix the patient's head and neck in the median supine position with the neck slightly flexed and rotated away from the side of puncture. A soft sponge should be placed underneath the neck. An 18G spinal needle is used to penetrate the postero-lateral aspect of the neck at the appropriate vertebral level using frequent AP and lateral X-rays or an image intensifier. The needle contacts the anterior surface of the transverse process and is then adjusted, preferably using an image intensifier, until it passes over the process and enters the foramen. Particular care must be taken to avoid penetrating the anterior compartment of the intervertebral foramen which contains the vertebral artery and vein. Radiofrequency or neurolytic techniques can be used. If the check lateral and AP X-rays are satisfactory a radiofrequency lesion is made by incremental steps or, after confirmation has been obtained by electrical stimulation, an alcohol injection can be made.

Thoracic

This may be performed with the patient prone with a pillow below the chest and the arms dependent but is often easier to do in the lateral position. The needle is introduced about 3–5 cm lateral to the midline of the spine and about 2 cm caudal to the chosen foramen. Local anaesthetic is injected as the needle advances. The needle is slowly advanced until at about 3 cm it touches bone usually the transverse process. Then further X-rays or image intensification are used to adjust the needle position. Thoracic rhizotomy is more difficult than cervical rhizotomy and the angle of insertion is steeper.

The patient often reports girdle pain as the needle enters the foramen. Aspiration should be made to ensure that the subarachnoid space or lung parenchyma has been penetrated. Before a lesion is made radiological information of needle position is essential and blood pressure should be maintained throughout the procedure.

Lumbar

Again, the lateral position is most convenient but if the prone position is preferred a pillow must be placed beneath the abdomen. The needle is inserted a little more lateral than for thoracic rhizotomy, about 6 cm from the midline and at the intervertebral foramenal level. Radicular pains are reported in the appropriate dermatomes when the nerve is contacted. Stimulation of the L1–L4 roots produces contraction of thigh muscles and L5–S2 stimulation produces leg and foot contraction. The needle tip penetrates over the posterior margin of the foramen in the rostral portion and lying on the medial border of the pedicle. Buttock paraesthesia and contraction of the anal sphincter is produced by S3–S5 stimulation. An alternative amd somewhat easier approach for the S1 root is to insert the needle in the midline at the lumbo-sacral interval directed a little laterally to the S1 root at the L5/S1 disc level.

Sacral

The patient is prone with a pillow beneath the pelvis. An 18G needle is inserted into each posterior sacral foramen aided by X-rays. S2, 3 and 4 can be individually destroyed by alcohol or radiofrequency. If S2 is to be preserved then the third, fourth or fifth roots can be destroyed by passing a needle through the sacral hiatus.

Open spinal rhizotomies are best performed by neurosurgeons and like all open procedures have the advantage of ease and precise identification which avoids injury to the motor roots. A simplified sacral rhizotomy can be performed by exposing the lumbo-sacral interval and performing a small laminectomy of the lower part of L5 and S1. The S2 root is identified and depending upon whether urinary function must be preserved a ligature is passed rostral or caudal to the root sleeve to encircle the dura. A second ligature is tied about 2 cm below the first. The dura and contained posterior and anterior roots are then sectioned and the wound closed in layers.

Spinal cord lesions

General

After entering the cord, fibres conveying pain and temperature synapse and relay within the dorsal horn and then cross the midline in the anterior commissure to enter the spinothalamic tract and ascend to the thalamus. The more medial fibres conveying vibration, touch and proprioception pass up the dorsal column on the same side of the cord to the brainstem.

A number of analgesic surgical procedures are available to deal with a wide variety of cancer pain syndromes. These include selective rhizotomy, where only pain fibres are selectively destroyed and fibres conveying normal sensation are preserved, and a number of stereo-tactic procedures including trigeminal tractotomy and nucleotomy and central cord lesions. Central cord lesions produce widespread analgesia but the technique is limited to centres with experience in special instrumentation.

All these procedures including percutaneous can only be performed by a surgeon with neurosurgical training and whenever possible cases requiring such treatment should be referred. Other practitioners would do best to confine themselves to peripheral procedures only.

Cordotomy (spino-thalamic tractotomy)

One of the oldest yet most effective of procedures, this is especially suitable for pain due to malignancy. Cordotomy has a high incidence of immediate relief although this steadily declines so that only 50% of survivors have satisfactory pain relief at 12 months post-operatively. Pain recurrence is often due to local extension or metastasis to areas outside the analgesic zone but allocheiria (reference of pain to the opposite side) does occur in pain due to pelvic lesions and can be troublesome.

The procedure can be performed at cervical or upper thoracic level but the cervical is safer and produces a higher analgesic level. It can be performed by an open procedure after cervical laminectomy or by percutaneous or stereotactic technique. An obvious hazard is damage to the cortico-spinal tract which lies just dorsal to the incision but other hazards are less obvious.

Close to the spino-thalamic fibres and deep to them lie autonomic fibres arranged somatotopically as a 'visceral spinal homunculus'. The fibres giving autonomic innervation to the diaphragm and intercostal muscles lie close to the cervical and thoracic portions of the spino-thalamic tract and can be injured by a deep incision. This has little importance unless the opposite respiratory apparatus is impaired or if ventilatory capacity is poor. Cordotomy may be performed for pain in the chest or arm due to bronchial cancer for which it is usually necessary to produce high analgesic levels by a *cervical cordotomy*.

Similarly micturition fibres are arranged close to the sacral fibres and in pain due to pelvic cancer with unilateral bladder involvement injury to this pathway whilst sectioning the sacral spino-thalamic fibres may result in urinary retention or incontinence.

In *thoracic cordotomy* there is obviously less risk of respiratory damage, since the diaphragmatic fibres have left the cord higher up, but high and sustained analgesic levels cannot always be produced.

Open cordotomy may be performed at cervical or thoracic levels. The advantage of cervical cordotomy is the ability to obtain high levels of analgesia and of course only cervical cordotomy is suitable for upper limb pain. Its main disadvantage is the risk of injury to respiratory fibres, although if the FEV_1 is more than 1.5 litres then in the absence of obvious respiratory distress the risk is small. Injury to the descending respiratory pathway as it lies close to the spino-thalamic tract reduces ipsilateral respiratory activity and if the contralateral respiratory apparatus is inadequate then only voluntary respiration is possible. The patient soon tires or becomes distressed and all too often the administration of opiates post-operatively to deal with this distress produces further respiratory depression and death.

With thoracic cordotomy on the other hand there is a greater risk of hemiparesis because of the greater cord manipulation needed within the more restricted space of the thoracic canal.

Percutaneous lateral cordotomy: This is performed at high cervical level by inserting laterally between C1 and C2 laminae a needle through which a sharp electrode passes to penetrate the anterior cord quadrant.

Although a relatively minor procedure its *long term* effectiveness has not been established and there are few follow-up reports for more than 6 months, although this is adequate for the vast majority of patients with cancer pain. By a relatively crude aiming technique and physiological stimulation a radiofrequency lesion is made within the quadrant. The initial success rate is nearly 90% and the mortality is low. The risk of paresis is higher than for open cordotomy in good hands with approximately 10% having weakness, reducing later to 8% who are, however, ambulant one month post-operatively. Respiratory complications are also high at nearly 9%.

In *percutaneous anterior cordotomy* the needle is introduced between C5 and C6 anteriorly through the disc. It is an easier technique than the C1, 2 lateral approach but initial aiming must be correct as the disc grasps the needle and prevents readjustment. It is a procedure,

however, worth considering if high levels of analgesia must be achieved
and damage to respiratory fibres must be avoided.

Stereotactic cordotomy: This technique requires specialized apparatus and expertise but because it is able to make a precise localised
lesion the complication rate is lower than for other open or percutaneous techniques (see Recommended Reading).

Percutaneous lateral cervical cordotomy

The procedure is carried out under general anaesthesia. The patient
lies supine with the neck held straight and slightly extended on a pillow
with a sponge beneath the neck. The Rosomoff kit provides all the
necessary instrumentation. Head holders are available which clamp
the skull between rubber pads but sandbags can be used and the head
can be fastened with strapping over the forehead

An image intensifier is valuable but if this is not available the head
and neck are placed over a cassette holder which will allow films to
be placed and removed without disturbing the patient's position. A
radiofrequency lesion generator which combines impedance and
stimulation instrumentation is essential. A special needle holder is
available commercially but is not essential. The essential instrumentation is an 18 gauge spinal needle through which an insulated
electrode passes whose tip is bared of insulation for 2 mm and is
sharpened. A simple stop is screwed into the electrode so that not
more than 4 mm can protrude beyond the needle. The 0.4 mm electrode
is either tungsten or stainless steel and can be insulated by polyethylene
tubing passed over it or by insulation paint. The indifferent electrode
(earth lead) is either a needle inserted into the ipsilateral deltoid or a
large electrode pad.

2–3 ml of 2% lignocaine is injected directly beneath the tip of the
mastoid process to a depth of approximately 3 cm.

The spinal needle is then pushed through the skin horizontally to
pass between the lamina of C1 and C2 and through the ligamentum
flavum until the dura is penetrated. Patients may complain of ear or
head pain if the C2 nerve root is contacted but a further small injection
of local anaesthetic at the site will usually prevent further distress.
Large amounts of local anaesthetic should not be injected because of
the risk of leakage or injection into the subarachnoid space producing
a high cervical block and temporary respiratory failure. If the needle's

passage is halted by bone an X-ray should be taken so that the angle can be adjusted.

When the subarachnoid space is penetrated cerebrospinal fluid will escape and 10 ml of air is then injected and an antero-posterior film taken through the open mouth and also a lateral X-ray. Water-soluble contrast media can be used instead of air but myodil is best avoided because of the risk of arachnoiditis.

The lateral X-ray should be inspected first. The needle tip should be directed to the anterior half of the cord. On the antero-posterior film the needle tip should lie close to, but not past, the edge of the odontoid. Without the use of a needle holder there is a tendency for the needle to be deviated in which case it must be held by hand or held by adhesive tape strapped to the patient's head whilst the electrode is passed down its lumen. The electrode is then locked into the needle and advanced towards the anterior quadrant. Impedance measurements are helpful in determining whether the electrode is within the cerebrospinal fluid where impedance is approximately 200 ohms. When the cord is contacted the impedance rises and when it enters the cord it becomes more than 600 ohms.

After cord contact the electrode is rapidly advanced into its substance. The arachnoid is tough and the electrode tip must be very sharp to prevent gross cord displacement. The patient often cries out when the cord is penetrated and reports a sensation in the opposite side of the body. The electrical leads are then clipped to the electrode and earth lead.

Electrical stimulation is now used, first at the low frequency of 2 Hz. With this frequency, at approximately 1–2 volts, there is contraction of ipsilateral neck muscles and trapezius but there should be no contraction of arm or leg since this would imply that the electrode was close to the corticospinal tract and was too posterior (Figure 29).

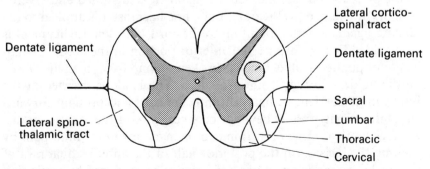

Figure 29 Cervical cord. Arrangement of spinothalamic tract

If this is the case the electrode should be withdrawn and replaced more anteriorly. When satisfactory responses to low stimulation are obtained higher frequencies (50–100 Hz) should be used but at lower voltages (less than 1 volt). Satisfactory electrode position has been obtained if the patient reports sensation in the opposite side of the body. Ipsilateral responses are almost invariably due to posterior placement in the posterior columns.

If stimulation results are satisfactory, radiofreqency coagulation should be performed. This is done either by using a standard current of approximately 50 mA and increasing the time in small increments up to 30–40 seconds, or by using a standard time of 30 seconds and increasing the current from 20 mA to 50 mA in small increments. The latter method is recommended. After each increment the contralateral pin prick sensation and ipsilateral power are tested and the coagulation continued until deep analgesia is produced without paresis.

Bilateral procedures are unwise because of the relatively imprecise nature of the procedure and the great risk of paresis and respiratory abnormality.

If the equipment for percutaneous radiofrequency cordotomy is not available, an open cordotomy operation should be performed.

Open high cervical cordotomy

The patient is positioned either prone or in the park bench position under endotracheal anaesthesia. The incision is midline from the occipital protruberance to about C5 and keeping strictly to the midline, the spines and lamina of C1, 2, 3 and 4 are exposed. (An experienced operator will find that a more limited exposure is adequate.) The arch of C1 is removed and the dura opened in the midline and sutured back to the muscles. The second dentate ligament is identified and severed from its attachment to the dura and a fine haemostat is applied to the dentate ligament with a point up to the cord. The dentate ligament is then folded back to expose the anterior portion of the cord. A 4 mm length of pointed scalpel blade is broken off and fixed in a pair of fine needle holders so that 2 mm protrudes. The blade is inserted at the insertion of the dentate ligament into the cord and brought forward circumferentially to just beyond the emergence of the anterior roots. A more limited selective section can be made for lower limb pain by limiting the incision in the posterior half of the anterior quadrant of the cord and a selective upper body analgesia produced by sectioning the anterior half. The occasional cordotomist is well advised to perform a conventional whole quadrant section. The dura and rest of the wound is closed in layers. Post-operatively the patient should not be given opiates because of the risk of respiratory distress and respiration should be carefully observed for the first 24 hours.

Neural stimulation

Neural stimulation either by dorsal column electrode placement or deep brain stimulation is limited to specialized centres and, because of the expense, fully implantable systems are generally used percutaneously with the electrode lead passing out through the skin. These have been left in place for many months but if life expectancy is good then totally implanted systems should be used.

Hypophysectomy

Hypophysectomy was introduced more than 30 years ago for the treatment of metastases in breast or prostatic cancer. Its aim then was to produce tumour regression but many patients were relieved of the pain of bony metastases without apparent effects upon tumour volume. The original technique of transcranial hypophysectomy has been supplanted by transnasal hypophysectomy. Chemical hypophysectomy by the trans-sphenoidal injection of alcohol into the sella has lately been advocated for all types of cancer pain, including many that are not hormone-dependent cancers. The best indication for hypophysectomy appears to be bone metastasis.

Both surgical and chemical hypophysectomies produce excellent pain relief but patients treated by chemical hypophysectomy frequently (about 50%) require a second procedure with a further 10% requiring a third procedure. The percutaneous and trans-sphenoidal aiming technique is not without hazard and trans-sphenoidal microscopic hypophysectomy is preferable if the expertise is available (see Recommended Reading).

Recommended reading

1. Bonica, J.J and Ventafridda, V. (eds.) (1979). *Advances in Pain Research and Therapy, Vol. 2. Pains and Advanced Cancer.* (New York: Raven Press)

2. Swerdlow, M. (ed.) (1986). *The Therapy of Pain,* 2nd Edn. (Lancaster: MTP Press)
3. White, J. C and Sweet W. H. (1969). *Pain and the Neurosurgeon. A Forty-Year Experience.* (Springfield, IL: Charles C. Thomas)

12

Symptom Control as it Relates to Pain Control

M. Baines

INTRODUCTION

Pain is the symptom most associated with cancer and most feared by patients and their families. However, other symptoms also commonly occur. Their control is essential in order to maintain a good quality of life for the cancer patient. The distress caused by persistent vomiting or dyspnoea, for example, can be as great as that caused by uncontrolled pain.

Even in a patient with far advanced cancer it is important to try to diagnose the cause of each symptom. Usually this can be determined by taking a careful history followed by a relevant physical examination. An exact diagnosis of the cause or causes of nausea, insomnia or confusion will often enable specific appropriate treatment to be instituted.

Sometimes a diagnosis cannot be made but an experienced doctor will know the likely cause of each symptom and the drugs most likely to ameliorate it.

In this chapter the common symptoms found in cancer patients will be examined with causative factors and appropriate treatment.

GASTROINTESTINAL SYMPTOMS

Dry or painful mouth

The following are the common causes seen in cancer patients:

(1) Drugs, especially phenothiazines, tricyclic antidepressants, antihistamines and cytotoxics,

(2) Oral candidosis,

(3) Dehydration,

(4) Oral tumours,

(5) Local radiotherapy.

Good oral hygiene is most important and will prevent many problems. Regular mouth washes should be given and some patients chew
gum or suck acid sweets or pineapple chunks to increase the flow of
saliva.

Dehydration should be corrected if it has been caused by a reversible
factor such as vomiting after chemotherapy or the development of an
operable intestinal obstruction. Rehydration using intravenous fluids
is not indicated in the terminally ill cancer patient. Fortunately the
only symptom of dehydration at this stage is a dry mouth and this
can be treated satisfactorily with local measures.

Oral candidosis is very common. It should be treated with nystatin
suspension (100 000 units/ml) 4-hourly. Dentures should be removed
and treated as well. Resistant cases often respond to a systemic anti-
fungal agent (e.g. ketoconazole 200 mg daily) if it is available.

Anorexia

A diminished desire for food is common in cancer patients and may be
the presenting symptom of the disease. Taste changes occur frequently;
often there is a dislike for meat or complaints that food tastes 'metallic'
or 'salty'. There are three treatment options:

Correction of causative factors

Nausea and vomiting, constipation, abdominal distension from ascites
and depression should be treated appropriately.

Dietary measures

Food should be attractively prepared and small portions served. Taste changes should be taken into account; many patients prefer a strong-tasting food to the traditional invalid fare.

In the early cancer patient it is reasonable to try to maintain a well balanced diet with adequate levels of protein, fibre, iron and vitamins. In those with anorexia due to advanced disease any enforced diet becomes an intolerable burden, and this should be explained to the family.

Glucocorticosteroids

These are the only effective drugs for treating anorexia and normally lead to an improvement in appetite within a week. The starting dose is prednisolone 15–30 mg daily or dexamethasone 2–4 mg daily. In patients with advanced disease this dose can usually be continued without causing side-effects. If the disease goes into remission the dose can be reduced or even stopped.

Dysphagia

When a patient complains of difficulty in swallowing it is important to identify which of the three stages of swallowing is affected:

(1)   Passing the bolus to the back of the throat,
(2)   Initiating the swallowing reflex,
(3)   Passage of the bolus down the oesophagus.

Careful questioning of the patient, observation of the act of swallowing and a knowledge of previous medical history will often point to the stage of swallowing affected and the cause of dysphagia.

In general dysphagia may be caused by painful lesions, mechanical obstruction or neuromuscular disorders. The common causes of dysphagia are:

Candidosis

This may spread from the mouth to the pharynx and oesophagus. If possible it should be treated with nystatin.

External pressure from tumours in the neck or mediastinum

Glucocorticosteroids (dexamethasone 6 mg/day) can lead to a temporary shinkage of tumour with improvement in symptoms. Steroids may also help the dysphagia caused by tumour infiltration of the muscles and nerves of the pharynx which can lead to a non-obstructive dysphagia from neuromuscular incoordination. Irradiation should be considered if available and if the patient is fit enough.

Oesophageal carcinoma

The insertion of an oesophageal tube or radiotherapy should always be considered if this is possible, because medication has little to offer.

If specific treatment for dysphagia is ineffective there are three other possibilities:

(1) Appropriate feeding,

(2) Nasogastric tube,

(3) Gastrostomy.

The choice of diet is a very individual matter but many cancer patients with dysphagia can be helped to find an appetising and nourishing diet in a liquid or semi-solid form. Most patients with severe dysphagia sooner or later develop an aspiration pneumonia which should be treated symptomatically.

Nausea and vomiting

These are caused by stimulation of the vomiting centres in the medulla oblongata in one or more ways:

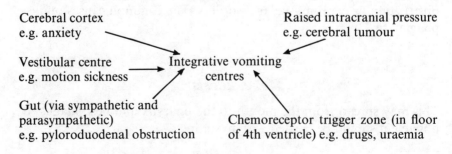

Cerebral cortex
e.g. anxiety

Raised intracranial pressure
e.g. cerebral tumour

Vestibular centre
e.g. motion sickness

Integrative vomiting
centres

Gut (via sympathetic and parasympathetic)
e.g. pyloroduodenal obstruction

Chemoreceptor trigger zone (in floor of 4th ventricle) e.g. drugs, uraemia

Diagnosis of the cause of vomiting in the cancer patient will often point to specific treatment being instituted. If this is not possible the most appropriate antiemetic drug can be chosen because the drugs available act at different sites (Table 9). Some diseases cause vomiting through more than one mechanism and combinations of antiemetic drugs acting at different sites may prove more effective than a single agent. Table 10 shows the causes of vomiting most commonly found in cancer patients.

Bearing in mind the mechanism of vomiting and the antiemetic drugs available, some of the common causes of vomiting are now discussed with suggested treatment.

Drug-induced vomiting

(1) Opiates, digoxin, and many chemotherapeutic agents have a direct effect on the chemoreceptor trigger zone. If it is not possible to discontinue the drug an antiemetic such as prochlorperazine should be given.

Table 9 Antiemetic drugs

Group	Examples	Dose/24 hours	Site of action
Phenothiazines	Chlorpromazine Prochlorperazine	50–150 mg 15–50 mg	Chemoreceptor trigger zone
Butyrophenones	Haloperidol	1.5–5 mg	Chemoreceptor trigger zone
Antihistamines	Promethazine	30–75 mg	Integrative vomiting centre
Anticholinergics	Hyoscine	0.4–0.6 mg single dose	
	Atropine	0.3–0.5 mg single dose	Integrative vomiting centre
Other	Metoclopramide	30–60 mg	Upper gut, increasing gastric peristalsis and relaxing pyloric antrum

Table 12 Causes of vomiting

Chemical causes
  Drugs
  Uraemia
  Hypercalcaemia
  Irradiation

Gastric causes
  Local irritation from drugs, blood, etc.
  External pressure
  Carcinoma of stomach
  Pyloroduodenal obstruction

Intestinal obstruction

Constipation

Raised intracranial pressure

Vestibular disturbance

Cough-induced vomiting

Psychogenic, especially anxiety

(2) Aspirin and other non-steroidal anti-inflammatory drugs (and alcohol) cause gastric irritation. Medication should be given with food or by suppository or a similar drug substituted with less gastrointestinal side-effects (see Chapter 7).

Uraemia

Uraemic vomiting can usually be controlled by antiemetics acting on the chemoreceptor trigger zone.

Hypercalcaemia

This may occur in the presence of widespread osteolytic bony metastases usually from primary tumours of breast, bronchus or myeloma. It can also occur in the absence of skeletal metastases and may be due to ectopic parathyroid hormone secreted by squamous carcinomas or carcinoma of the kidney.

The symptoms of hypercalcaemia are usually described as weakness, anorexia, nausea and vomiting leading to drowsiness, confusion and coma. However, this progression is not often seen; the patient may present with confusion without preceding vomiting and the severity of symptoms does not correlate well with the corrected calcium level.

Mild hypercalcaemia (under 3 mol/1) will usually respond to steroids alone. If the patient is vomiting, an injection of hydrocortisone 100 mg should be given followed by oral prednisolone 30 mg daily. Other treatments include encouraging oral fluids plus a loop diuretic such as frusemide and oral phosphate 1–3 g daily.

In cancer patients with very advanced disease the development of severe hypercalcaemia (over 3 mol/1) should be considered a terminal event and only treated symptomatically.

Raised intracranial pressure

This is an unusual cause of vomiting but may occur with primary or secondary cerebral tumours. Treatment is with corticosteroids, using dexamethasone 16 mg daily and urgent consideration of surgery or radiotherapy if available. If these are not indicated the steroid dose should be reduced to the lowest level compatible with symptom control. If steroids are not used, vomiting can usually be well controlled with an antiemetic.

Gastric causes

(1) External pressure from hepatomegaly causes early satiation with flatulence, hiccup and vomiting. Treatment is with metoclopramide 10 mg before meals and a defoaming agent such as dimethicone.

(2) Intrinsic involvement of the stomach from carcinoma, including linitis plastica, often causes severe vomiting. Treatment is not very satisfactory but metoclopramide may help. Glucocorticosteroids sometimes give temporary relief (see p. 158).

(3) Pyloroduodenal obstruction occurs with carcinoma of the stomach or pancreas. The patient should be considered for palliative surgery (see Chapter 9). If this is not possible the vomiting is difficult to manage medically. Metoclopramide is usually

ineffective and a nasogastric tube may be more distressing than the vomiting itself. However, a proportion of these patients respond temporarily to high dose steroids given on the assumption that the symptoms were caused by tumour plus surrounding inflammatory oedema. Dexamethasone 6–8 mg daily should be given by injection at first. If there is no response in 3–4 days, the dose should be stopped; if effective it can be continued orally.

Intestinal obstruction

A proportion of patients with gynaecological and large bowel malignancies develop intestinal obstruction. Ovarian carcinoma is the commonest cause and 25% of patients with this disease will obstruct. The obstruction may be complete or incomplete (subacute). It may be caused by narrowing of the lumen or disordered gut motility due to tumour in mesentery or gut muscle. There may be a single site but frequently multiple sites in ileum and colon are involved.

Each cancer patient who develops intestinal obstruction should be considered for palliative surgery if available and if he is fit enough. Unfortunately results of surgery are poor; in those with advanced disease, operative mortality is high and symptoms commonly persist.

It is nearly always possible to control pain in an obstructed patient by the use of an antispasmodic drug such as hyoscine for colic and an opiate analgesic such as morphine for other visceral pain. A coeliac plexus block (see p. 122) should also be considered. It is not always possible to control vomiting but it can usually be greatly improved with a lessening of nausea (which patients find worse than vomiting) and a diminution of vomits to once or twice a day The most useful drugs are prochlorperazine 5–10 mg three times daily or chlorpromazine 25–100 mg three times daily. These can be given orally, by injection or by suppository, if available.

Hiccup

This may occur in uraemia, in diseases affecting the stomach or diaphragm and occasionally with cerebral tumours. Holding the breath or rebreathing into a paper bag (which increases pCO_2) may give relief. The two most effective drugs are metoclopramide 10 mg and chlorpromazine 25 mg. They can be given when required for occasional bouts of hiccup or three times a day if the symptom persists. A severe and distressing episode may respond to chlorpromazine 25 mg i.v. or hyoscine 0.4 mg i.v.

Constipation

This is a very common problem for the cancer patient and causes more anxiety than almost any other symptom. There are many predisposing factors:

(1)   Poor appetite,

(2)   Diet low in roughage,

(3)   Inactivity,

(4)   Dehydration due to fever and vomiting,

(5)   Drugs such as narcotic analgesics, tricyclic antidepressants and phenothiazines.

Unfortunately many of these factors are difficult to alter though an attempt can be made to increase fibre in the diet and encourage mobility; corticosteroids can be given to the patient with advanced disease to improve appetite.

The practical management of a patient with constipation depends on the physical findings, especially on rectal examination.

Three situations commonly arise:

(1)   The rectum is loaded with hard faeces. Evacuation from below is required using either suppositories or a phosphate enema; if these are ineffective a manual removal may be needed. An oil retention enema should be given, at night, if faecal masses are too large to pass without causing pain.

(2)   The rectum is loaded with soft faeces. If there is discomfort, suppositories or a phosphate enema should be given; if there is no discomfort the condition can be treated with laxatives.

(3)   The rectum is empty but faecal masses can be palpated abdominally. Treatment is with laxatives.

Laxatives must be used following rectal measures and they should be given routinely after starting narcotic analgesia. There are two main types of laxatives:

Faecal softeners – These include methyl cellulose and magnesium sulphate which take up water and thus increase the volume of intestinal contents, and liquid paraffin which is minimally absorbed and thus softens and lubricates.

Stimulant purgatives – These increase peristalsis in the colon. They include senna and phenolphthalein.

Persistent constipation is best managed with a combination of both types of aperient. This will avoid either painful colic or a bowel loaded with soft faeces, problems which can arise if a stimulant or softening aperient is given alone. The choice will depend on local availability and there are a number of convenient combined preparations. The dose should be gradually increased until a regular soft bowel action is obtained.

Occasionally, in spite of regular aperients, the bowels do not open regularly and a good general rule is for a rectal examination to be performed on the third day, inserting suppositories if the rectum is loaded. Such a regime will avoid the physical and mental distress of patients who are constipated for a week or more.

RESPIRATORY SYMPTOMS

Dyspnoea

Dyspnoea may be defined as a distressing difficulty in breathing; it is therefore subjective (what the patient feels). Hyperventilation (noted by the doctor) consists of tachypnoea (rapid breathing) and hyperpnoea (increased depth of respiration).

Dyspnoea is a common symptom in cancer patients and is found in 65–70% of those with advanced lung cancer.

Mechanism

The respiratory centre in the brainstem can be stimulated chemically by a raised pCO_2, a lowered pO_2, or a raised pH. It can also be stimulated by afferent impulses from the lungs, notably the juxtapulmonary receptors and lung irritant receptors.

Causes of dyspnoea

The following are commonly found in the cancer patient:

(1) Malignant lung disease
     Carcinoma of bronchus
     Pulmonary metastases
     Pleural effusion
     Lymphangitis carcinomatosa.

(2) Non-malignant lung disease
     Chronic obstructive airways disease
     Pulmonary oedema due to heart failure
     Asthma
     Pneumonia
     Pulmonary fibrosis (sometimes postradiotherapy).

(3) Other diseases
     Anaemia
     Uraemia
     Ascites.

(4) Anxiety.

   In practice dyspnoea is usually multifactorial, for example a patient
with longstanding chronic obstructive airways disease who develops
a bronchial carcinoma with a small pleural effusion and who is very
anxious.

Treatment

An attempt should be made to diagnose the cause (or causes) of
dyspnoea. Heart failure should be treated with diuretics and digoxin,
bronchospasm with bronchodilators, pneumonia with antibiotics and
physiotherapy.
   Specific anticancer treatment should be used if available, radiotherapy for mediastinal glands, hormonal manipulation for metastases
from breast carcinoma, chemotherapy for responsive tumours.
   However, the time comes with most dyspnoeic cancer patients when
specific treatment no longer helps; the effusion rapidly reaccumulates
after aspiration, pneumonia no longer responds to antibiotics, the
tumour enlarges. At this stage the aim must be to relieve the symptom
rather than alter the progress of the disease.

There are four treatment options – oxygen, opiates, tranquillizers or hyoscine.

Oxygen – In chronic dyspnoea due to malignant disease better control is obtained with the use of opiates and other drugs than with oxygen.

Opiates – These affect respiration in several ways:

(1)   Reduce sensitivity of the respiratory centre to raised pCO_2 or lowered pO_2.

(2)   Reduce sensation of dyspnoea.

(3)   Reduce pain and anxiety.

In practice dyspnoeic patients have less respiratory distress. There may also be an improved capacity to exercise due to a reduction in respiratory overdrive which occurs in atelectasis and in anxiety.

The starting dose of oral opiate should be low, corresponding to 2.5–5 mg morphine 4-hourly, increasing slowly if necessary. Lower doses of opiates are needed to control dyspnoea than to control pain. The common fear is that opiates inevitably cause severe respiratory depression if given to a dyspnoeic patient. This is not true if the dose is titrated carefully.

Tranquillizers – Diazepam and other benzodiazepines are sometimes used to control dyspnoea; the dose is diazepam 2 mg three times daily or 10 mg at night. The effect is probably due to their anxiolytic and muscle relaxant properties.

The anxiety of the dyspnoeic patient can also be treated with relaxation techniques and with counselling, refuting the common fear of suffocating or of choking to death.

Hyoscine – This anticholinergic drug has the following actions:

(1)   It dries up glandular secretions.

(2)   It relaxes smooth muscle.

(3)   It is a central sedative (unlike atropine which is a central stimulant).

It is widely used to abolish the so-called 'Death rattle' which occurs in dying patients unable to cough up bronchial secretions and is distressing to the watching family – if not to the patient himself.

The dose is 0.4–0.6 mg by injection and it is given with morphine 5–10 mg. This is added to reduce dyspnoea further and to prevent the occasional agitation from hyoscine.

COUGH

Mechanism

Coughing is caused by stimulation of the cough centre in the medulla by afferent impulses from the upper or lower respiratory tract.

A *dry cough* is usually caused by pressure on a bronchus by primary or metastatic tumour. It also occurs in the mucosal inflammation stage of acute bronchitis and it is exacerbated by the inhalation of dry air and smoke.

A *productive cough* results in the expectoration of mucus which may or may not be infected. It is caused by chronic bronchitis, lung abscess, pneumonia or tumour with secondary infection. Pulmonary oedema due to heart failure causes white, frothy sputum.

Treatment

The cause of cough should be identified, if possible, and specific treatment offered – for example antibiotics for a chest infection and palliative radiotherapy for a tumour. However, in many cases such treatment is not possible, or is ineffective, and symptomatic relief is required. In general terms it is reasonable to suppress a dry cough but a productive cough should be allowed to continue unless it is disturbing sleep or the patient is too weak to expectorate effectively.

Agents which relieve cough may act peripherally on the respiratory tract, or centrally on the cough centre in the medulla.

Peripheral action

(1)   On inspired air. The inspiration of warm, moist air will often relieve a distressing cough and this can be achieved with a steam kettle, humidifier or the use of benzoin inhalations.

(2)   On bronchial secretions. Expectorants such as ammonium chloride and ipecacuanha are gastric irritants and may lead to vomiting. Mucolytics reduce the viscosity of bronchial secretions by interfering with the synthesis of mucus or increasing its breakdown. They can be given orally as bromhexine. The oral route is acceptable and has been shown to be effective and is used if the patient finds expectoration difficult.

Central action

(1) Codeine and pholcodeine. These are often effective if given in adequate doses, codeine 30–60 mg 4-hourly.

(2) An opiate is often required to control the distressing cough of a patient with a bronchial carcinoma. The starting dose should correspond to morphine 5 mg 4-hourly; this can be increased as necessary to control the symptom.

URINARY SYMPTOMS

Urinary frequency and incontinence

These symptoms may occur early in the cancer patient whose disease affects the pelvis or central nervous system. They are commonly found later in the debilitated patient with advanced disease. For the following causes there is specific treatment.

(1) In urinary tract infection the urine should be cultured, if possible, and an appropriate antibiotic given.

(2) Pelvic tumours may be reduced in size following radiotherapy.

(3) Polyuria from diabetes mellitus or diabetes insipidus requires appropriate treatment.

(4) Treatment for spinal metastases leading to compression of the spinal cord or cauda equina is with dexamethasone 30 mg daily (followed by urgent radiotherapy or decompression laminectomy if possible).

Unfortunately the most common causes are not amenable to specific treatment but the following symptomatic measures should be considered.

(1) Anticholinergic drugs are used in urinary frequency because they increase the volume of the bladder at which the first desire to micturate is experienced.

(2) A urinary condom is useful for nocturnal incontinence but is not often tolerated throughout the 24 hours for more than a few days.

(3) A catheter is usually the best way of treating severe frequency or incontinence. A self-retaining catheter should be passed under

full aseptic conditions; in most patients this is quite painless. If catheterization is expected to be difficult due, for example, to a large vulval carcinoma or to considerable anxiety, it is helpful to give intravenous diazepam a few minutes beforehand.

It is impossible to maintain a sterile urine in a catheterized patient and long-term antibiotics have no place as resistance occurs. Infections are only treated if they are symptomatic; if they occur frequently a urinary antiseptic such as hexamine hippurate 1 g twice daily will often prevent them. Daily bladder washouts with chlorhexidine are used if there is a lot of sediment which could cause catheter blockage.

Urinary retention

The commonest cause of retention in the debilitated cancer patient is constipation. It can also be caused by bladder neck or urethral obstruction, neurological problems and by drugs, especially tricyclic antidepressants, phenothiazine and anticholinergics.

Haematuria

Slight haematuria can occur with a urinary infection but significant haematuria is usually caused by a malignancy involving the urinary tract or occasionally by trauma associated with catherization.

Radiotherapy if available should be considered for a carcinoma involving the bladder if the patient is well enough and has not been fully irradiated. Clot retention should be treated with catheterization and citrate bladder washouts. Persistent haematuria is sometimes eased by an antifibrinolytic drug such as aminocaproic acid.

Fistulae

A proportion of patients with pelvic malignancies develop fistulae. These rarely occur unless pelvic irradiation has been given and the risk of fistula formation often deters the radiotherapist from treating or re-treating this area.

Vesicovaginal fistula

The resulting incontinence can often be managed with the use of a large size indwelling catheter with or without vaginal tampons.

Rectovesical or colovesical fistulae

A palliative colostomy should be considered as the presence of faecal material in the bladder causes severe pain.

Rectovaginal fistulae

The only satisfactory treatment is a palliative colostomy.

It is occasionally impossible to prevent faecal or urinary incontinence. In these cases it remains important to minimize perineal excoriation and also unpleasant odours. Regular cleansing and changes of dressing are required, with the use of a barrier cream and one of the many deodorants available.

SKIN PROBLEMS

Pruritus

Many cancer patients have a dry skin and this may cause a mild irritation. Treatment involves avoiding soap and using an emulsifying ointment in the bath. Crotamiton cream is a mild antipruritic; antihistamine creams should be avoided as they can cause dermatitis. Antihistamines can be given orally; their benefit is probably due to the mild sedation they cause.

Patients with obstructive jaundice can develop severe pruritus due to the accumulation of bile salts.

Fungating tumours

Breast cancer is by far the commonest malignancy to cause fungation but it can occur with a great variety of other tumours. Such an outward manifestation of disease is always distressing to the patient due to the altered body image it causes and to problems from leakage and smell.

Radiotherapy, chemotherapy and hormonal manipulation should be used if appropriate and available.

Regular cleansing of the lesion is important, at least daily. The value of local applications is to prevent the dressing from sticking and to reduce secondary infection which is the cause of malodour. An emulsion of liquid paraffin and 4% povidone–iodine in a ratio of 4:1 has been found effective. It is used to clean the wound and then gauze soaked in it is applied as a dressing.

If there is a persistent capillary bleeding from the tumour a non-adherent dressing should be applied and covered with gauze soaked in 1 in 1000 adrenaline.

Vulval lesions should be treated with frequent washdowns with a mild antiseptic such as chlorhexidine 1 in 2000.

Occasionally despite these measures there are persistent problems with smell. This is usually due to secondary anaerobic infection and can be treated appropriately.

NEUROPSYCHOLOGICAL SYMPTOMS

Insomnia

Many patients with malignant disease sleep poorly due to unrelieved physical or mental distress. Before prescribing a hypnotic it is necessary to enquire if sleep is disturbed by pain, night sweats, fear of incontinence or other physical symptoms for which appropriate relief can be given. More often anxiety, depression or a fear of dying in the night prevent normal sleep; a careful enquiry will usually uncover these and they can be helped both by counselling and by psychotropic drugs.

If hypnotics are required it is important to bear in mind the duration of action of the various hypnotic agents. A short acting drug (e.g. temazepam) will give little risk of daytime sedation. However, in anxious patients in whom some daytime sedation is required it would be an advantage to use a longer acting hypnotic (e.g. nitrazepam).

Care should be taken in prescribing hypnotics for the elderly because they may cause or increase confusion.

Night sweats are an occasional cause of insomnia; they often respond to indomethacin given as a suppository, or as a sustained-relief tablet at night.

Confusion

The differential diagnosis and treatment of confusion are two of the most difficult problems facing the doctor who cares for cancer patients.

Whereas pain or perhaps incontinence is the symptom most dreaded by the patient himself, confusion is probably the symptom which most hurts the family.

In order to find the cause of confusion the following steps are suggested.

(1)   Medical history: ask if the confusion developed rapidly or slowly, whether it followed a change in medication or environment, if it is associated with severe anxiety or depression.

(2)   Clinical examination: note especially any neurological signs, evidence of sepsis, possibility of anaemia or cardiac failure which could lead to cerebral anoxia.

(3)   Full blood count and biochemical profile if possible.

Such steps will usually lead to a clinical diagnosis being made and this may be all that is practicable in the patient with advanced disease.

The following causes of confusion are commonly seen; often two or more are found:

(1)   Drug induced, especially due to psychotropic drugs, narcotic analgesics or alcohol,

(2)   Infections, especially in the chest or urinary tract,

(3)   Biochemical disturbance such as hypercalcaemia or uraemia,

(4)   Cerebral anoxia,

(5)   Cerebral tumours, primary or secondary,

(6)   Cerebrovascular disease,

(7)   Psychogenic, severe anxiety or depression and, in the elderly, an altered environment.

From such a list, it is apparent that specific treatment can be given in a proportion of cases, chest infection treated, sedation reduced and hypercalcaemia corrected. Even if the underlying cause cannot be corrected it is a great help to the family to know that the confusion is caused by physical disease rather than insanity.

Psychotropic drugs have only a minor place in the management of a confused patient; they cannot restore mental function deranged by disease but may make a restless and aggressive patient easier to manage. Haloperidol 5–10 mg by injection is useful in an emergency followed by 5–10 mg daily by mouth in divided doses. Chlorpromazine 50–100 mg immediately followed by 50–100 mg daily is useful if extra sedation is required.

Weakness

This is the commonest symptom of the patient with advanced cancer but it can also be the presenting symptom of treatable disease.

The complaint of 'weakness' is often poorly correlated with any measurable loss of strength and is obviously related to the patient's expectations of himself as well as his present physical situation. There are those with incurable and advancing disease who complain of increasing weakness and request help for this. Sometimes, even at this stage, there is a correctable factor such as secondary infection, hypercalcaemia or hypokalaemia which require specific treatment. Five other options remain:

(1) Glucocorticosteroids – Prednisolone 15–30 mg/day will usually lead to an improvement both in appetite and general sense of wellbeing. It is an invaluable treatment for many with advanced cancer; if the disease progresses more slowly than expected or side-effects become a problem the dose can be reduced.

(2) Blood transfusions, if available, may help if lethargy is associated with other symptoms of anaemia but are often disappointing for the treatment of weakness alone, probably because weakness has so many causes. It is meddlesome to treat a low haemoglobin in a symptom-free patient unless further treatment such as chemotherapy or radiotherapy is planned.

(3) Antidepressants – clinical depression, or far more often the natural sadness of the patient with cancer, is sometimes expressed as a complaint of weakness. This should be treated with emotional

support to the patient and family and occasionally with anti-depressant drugs.

(4) Physiotherapy.

(5) Acceptance and adjustment.

As the disease progresses there is an almost inevitable decline in strength. This can only be coped wtih satisfactorily if it is accepted and the pattern of daily life suitably modified with the cultivation of less active pursuits. The company of family and friends, a short outing, a good book can all continue to bring great pleasure.

Recommended reading

1. Saunders, C.M. (ed.) (1984). *The Management of Terminal Disease*. (London: Edward Arnold)
2. Twycross, R. G. and Lack S. A. (1984). *Therapeutics in Terminal Care*. (London: Pitman)

PART FOUR
Terminal Care

13

Terminal Care: Organization and Technical Aspects

R. G. Twycross

The aim of terminal care is to help the patient, despite the cancer and increasing physical limitations, to go on having a good quality of life until he dies. We undertake this against a background of his illness, his symptoms, his fears, his frustrations, his family, his friends, his cultural background, his beliefs and his ability or inability to accept what is happening. Care of the dying cancer patient should be approached positively, but the doctor, nurses and others involved should not underestimate the problems they face. Good terminal care is hard work, often very hard work, though perhaps all the more rewarding for this.

Care of the dying extends far beyond pain relief and the alleviation of other symptoms – important though these are. It includes supporting the patient emotionally as he adjusts to his decreasing physical ability and as he mourns in anticipation the loss of his family, his friends and his hopes for the future. It also includes supporting the family as they adjust to the fact that one of them is dying.

FEAR OF DEATH

Most humans fear death; it is part of the survival instinct. People feel unease in life-threatening situations. Unease is also felt in the presence

173

of death because it evokes fear about one's own future death. There is, therefore, a natural tendency to withdraw from the dying. In addition, there is a cultural factor, a collective fear of death. In every society, whether primitive or sophisticated, the corporate fear of death is focused on one or two particular diseases, or a group of diseases. Cancer is more feared than most other diseases – despite the fact that up to 40% of cancer sufferers can now be cured. The doctor's instinctive reaction to cancer is equally exaggerated. More than with most other conditions, a feeling of helplessness may creep in.

Some doctors find themselves unable to care for the dying patient at all; others continue on only a very superficial level. Death is seen as the ultimate disaster, and terminal care becomes a kind of macabre play in which the patient is 'jollied' along until the final curtain falls.

The care of the dying patient and his family is one of the more demanding of the doctor's responsibilities. It is also one of the most rewarding. Yet because he feels powerless in the face of the relentless advancing disease, the doctor's ability to help may become neutered. It is, however, possible for the doctor to overcome his negative feelings and so continue to help the dying patient and his family.

TEAMWORK

Terminal care comprises:

(1)   Relief of pain and other symptoms,

(2)   Psychological support of the patient,

(3)   Psychological support of the family.

All three compoments are vital to the whole and if one part is neglected it seriously hampers progress in the other two. Terminal care cannot be administered by any one individual; it calls for a group of individuals working together as a 'team'. The composition of the team may vary but includes the patient himself, the immediate family, friends, doctor, and nurses. The team is collectively concerned for the total wellbeing of the patient and the family – physical, psychological, spiritual and social.

Moreover, unless the nurses, and at home the family, actively participate in symptom control, the lead given by the doctor will be seriously undermined. The nurses must:

(1)   Give the patient opportunity to express anxieties and fears.

(2)   Encourage the patient by quietly emphasizing that his symp-
      tom(s) will soon be better controlled.

(3)   Advise about diet and fluid intake.

(4)   Contact the doctor if the patient fails to get a good night's sleep.

(5)   Contact the doctor rather than wait for his next visit if the patient
      becomes less well when a new treatment is started.

(6)   Advise the patient when to increase the dose of analgesic.

(7)   Support the patient through the period of initial side-effects
      commonly seen with morphine-like drugs.

Without this degree of involvement, the doctor's task is made considerably more difficult and occasionally impossible. On the other
hand, a nurse is unlikely to feel happy involving herself in these ways
unless she is encouraged to by the doctor.

   It is necessary, therefore, for doctors and nurses to establish a
common baseline of intent in relation to the terminally ill. From this
foundation, enriched by mutual trust and respect, the possibility of
good terminal care emerges.

COMMUNICATION

At a time of increasing uncertainty the patient wants to hear two
things from the doctor:

(1)   'No matter what happens to you I am going to do all I can to
      help you.'

(2)   'You may have cancer, you may be dying, but you are still
      important to me.'

Only part of this can be said in words: this fundamental message of
support and companionship is conveyed to the patient largely by
means of non-verbal communication.

ADJUSTING TO A POOR PROGNOSIS

People cope with crises in life by using a variety of defence or coping
mechanisms. These enable them to continue to function without

excessive anxiety, depression or anger, and allow them time to adapt to the new situation. Common defence mechanisms include denial, displacement, regression, intellectualization and religious faith.

In the dying patient the commonest defence mechanism is probably denial. Denial basically implies obliteration or minimization of reality by ignoring it. It may, however, be associated with evidence of anxiety.

As denial gives way to other methods of coping, there may be episodes of anger, anxiety and depression. The care givers around the patient need to recognize these as part of the process of adjustment so that they themselves do not become angry and frustrated. It should be noted that adjustment to a poor prognosis takes time, and that different coping mechanisms are employed by different patients. At first patients do not generally cope well with 'naked' truth. The initial blow may be softened by stressing what medical science has to offer, erring on the side of optimism. Patients show the greatest confidence in doctors who combine realism with optimism.

Most patients adapt to the fact that they have a limited prognosis and they try to make the best of their situation. Some become positively resigned, and this casts a shadow of gloom across the final phase of the patient's illness. A minority refuse to accept the prognosis and continue to be aggressive and angry. This is perhaps the most maladaptive of all psychological postures, and the most distressing for the family and those caring for the patient. The majority of dying patients, however, show great fortitude. This encourages the doctor and provides the emotional resources for dealing with more difficult situations.

Few patients talk to a doctor about their fears, particularly the more diffuse, less well defined fear of death. This may be because of doctor's lack of time, though many doctors convey the impression of being unwilling to communicate at this level. Given an unhurried atmosphere and the doctor's willingness to discuss such matters, many patients appreciate being able to talk. Gentle, sympathetic and gradual communication of the truth – within the context of continued support and encouragement – does much to restore and maintain hope.

APPROPRIATE TREATMENT

In terminal illness the primary aim is no longer to preserve life but to make the life that remains as comfortable and as meaningful as possible. Thus, what may be appropriate treatment in an acutely ill patient may be inappropriate in the dying. Cardiac resuscitation, artificial respiration, intravenous infusion, nasogastric tubes, and antibiotics are all primarily supportive measures for use in acute or acute-on-chronic illnesses to assist a patient through the initial period towards recovery of health. To use such measures in a patient who is clearly close to death and has no expectancy of a return to health is generally inappropriate, and is therefore bad medicine. We have no right or duty, legal or ethical, to prescribe a lingering death. It is a question therefore of what is appropriate treatment from a biological point of view in the light of the patient's personal and social circumstances.

Physical therapy is part of medical care even in the dying. Eventually, however, rehabilitation becomes impossible and the patient is encouraged to remain in bed. On the other hand, many dying patients are unnecessarily restricted, often by cautious relatives, even though they are capable of a greater degree of activity and independence. The patient's potential will be realized, however, only if troublesome symptoms are controlled and gentle encouragement is given by an attentive doctor. Unfortunately, through lack of instruction, many doctors feel inadequate in this area of care and are unaware of the therapeutic possibilities that currently exist in relation to symptom control (see Chapter 14).

SYMPTOMATIC TREATMENT

Pain is not a constant feature of terminal cancer, nor is it the only symptom patients experience. Because of the importance of the subject the principles underlying symptom control are re-emphasized here to supplement the detailed description of symptom control given in Chapter 12.

Most symptoms are caused by multiple factors. It is a case of recognizing the various contributory factors and then 'chipping' away at them. In this way, although the principal pathological process remains unaltered, it is generally possible to relieve the patient's symptoms either completely or to a considerable extent.

Explain in simple terms the underlying mechanism(s). For example: 'The shortness of breath is partly due to the illness itself and partly due to fluid at the base of the right lung. In addition, there is some degree of 'water-logging' throughout the body, particularly in the lungs, and you are slightly anaemic – people with your sort of illness tend to be. We cannot wave a magic wand and get rid of the underlying tumour – you know that – but this is what we are going to do about the extra fluid . . .'.

The fact that the doctor is able to demonstrate that he understands the causes of a particular symptom is reassuring to the patient. No longer is his condition shrouded in mystery – the doctor understands.

Discuss treatment options with the patient and, if possible, decide together on the immediate course of action. Few things are more demeaning to a person's self-esteem than to be disregarded in discussion concerning treatment options. It is hurtful when a doctor ignores the patient and treats him as an imbecile.

Explain the treatment to the relatives. Discussion with the family is of secondary importance from the patient's point of view. The dying have a right to be treated as what they usually are: sane, sensible adults. However, it is essential to explain the proposed treatment to the relatives. This is particularly important when the patient is at home, and the family members are helping with care.

Do not limit treatment to the use of drugs. For example, pruritus can be relieved in the majority of patients without resort to antihistamine drugs. A simple hand cream applied to dry, itching skin several times a day and soap eliminated in favour of emulsifying ointment are frequently sufficient.

Prescribe drugs prophylactically for persistent symptoms.

Seek a colleague's advice in seemingly intractable situations.

Never say 'I have tried everything' or 'There is nothing more I can do'. It is possible to develop a repertoire of alternative measures. It is also important to reassure the patient that you, the doctor, are going to stand by him and do all you can.

SIMPLE PHYSICAL MEASURES

Exercise seems the natural antidote to weakness and many patients welcome the suggestion of physiotherapy aided by trained staff, the nursing team or the family (Table 11). Undoubtedly patients benefit, both mentally and physically, from keeping active as long as possible.

In bedridden patients a pillow under the knees and one behind the back will help prevent or ease back pain. To prevent stiffness or pain occurring in the joints these should be exercised both actively and passively as fully as possible, two or three times a day. For example, after mastectomy the patient may be unwilling to move the shoulder or arm because of pain. In this circumstance, exercises are invaluable.

Table 11   Physical therapies

Therapy of muscle spasm	Massage Cold and/or heat Collars, traction Passive exercises Chair/bed positioning
Counter-irritation	Mentholated ointments Heat or cold Pressure, vibration, rubbing
Mobilization	Exercises to strengthen and prevent contractures and spasm Aids for walking, (walkers, crutches, canes)
Immobilization	Teach techniques to avoid strain or fatigue Aids – collars, corsets, splints, slings, traction
General relaxation	Breathing exercises Distraction Prayer/meditation Hypnosis

Bedsores

Cachectic and immobile patients run a considerable risk of developing pressure sores. This risk is greatly increased if the patient is paraplegic, incontinent or can lie comfortably only in one position. Prevention is the aim and this will involve regular turning and gentle rubbing of the affected area by a nurse or one of the family. The application of a semipermeable membrane dressing such as Opsite (if available) will prevent the shearing forces between skin and bedclothes which accelerate the formation of bedsores. Once a sore has developed the avoidance of pressure is even more important.

Splintage

When spinal and/or limb movement is very painful (for example, pathological fracture of a vertebra) a rigid spinal support may give

greater relief. When there are weak or paralysed joints, suitable splinting can give support and prevent deformity. If commercial splints are
not available, a practical splint can be made from plaster of Paris,
wood or even cardboard.

Relaxation and Massage

Some body pains are due to muscle tension and can be relieved by
teaching the patient how to relax the tense muscles in the affected
area. Massage can reduce pain for several hours. It can be carried
out by one of the family. Light massage also helps the patient to relax.
Firmer tissue-moving massage helps to stimulate lymphatic circulation. This should begin on the trunk to open up normal lymphatic
channels. Moving distally along the affected limb, the masseur seeks
to open up lymph channels sequentially, allowing lymph to empty
proximally into the areas already stimulated.

Stomas

There are a number of problems which can occur when a stoma is
formed on the body surface after colostomy, ileostomy, ureterostomy,
etc. The skin around the stoma becomes irritated and painful and
this often creates additional psychological problems. Careful daily
cleansing of the skin with a simple salt solution or even clean water
will be helpful. If non-irritating stoma bags are available these should
be used. In the case of painful constipation in a patient with a
colostomy, benefit may be obtained by irrigating the colon with about
1 litre of water, daily if necessary, while an appropriate oral laxative
regimen is being introduced.

CARE OF THE FAMILY

The care of the family is an integral part of the care of the dying.
A contented family increases the likelihood of a contented patient.
Relative–doctor communication generally needs to be initiated and
maintained by the doctor. It is easy to neglect the relatives because
they are reluctant to bother the doctor 'as he is so busy'. There is
much to be said, at the time of diagnosis and later, for joint interviews –

patient, spouse, and doctor. The doctor should also make an opportunity to see both the patient and the close relatives on their own.
Further separate or joint interviews can then be arranged as necessary.

As with the patient, it is not generally necessary or wise to tell the
family the whole truth (as you see it) at one time. If the family
and patient are too far 'out of step' regarding knowledge about the
diagnosis and prognosis, it can create a barrier between them. A
common initial reaction is 'You won't tell him, will you, doctor?' or
'We'd prefer you not to tell him, doctor'. This should be seen as the
initial shock reaction and not as an excuse for saying nothing to the
patient.

If the family and patient are to be mutually supportive, it is
necessary to help all concerned to be more open with each other. It
is important to remember that the family cannot forbid the doctor
from discussing the diagnosis and prognosis with the patient.

Admission to hospital may be seen as a defeat by the family. It is
necessary to emphasize that you are surprised they managed to cope
for so long and that now, with the need for day and night care, it is
impossible for one (or two) people to continue to cope alone without
a break. Frequent visits should be encouraged, if practical. Separation
anxiety may be reduced by encouraging them to help in the care of
the patient – adjusting pillows, refilling a water jug, helping with a
blanket bath and assisting at mealtimes. Some relatives need to be
taught how to visit, to behave as they would at home, e.g. sit and read
a book or newspaper, knit, watch the television together. It should
be emphasized that they do not have to keep up an exhausting conversation about trivia.

A proportion of patients with terminal illness improve following
admission as a result of the control of pain and other symptoms. They
become physically independent again and no longer need to be in
hospital. Many relatives have fears about what will happen should
the patient be discharged from hospital. A trial day out or weekend
at home does much to allay their fears or it may confirm that discharge
is impractical. Clear advice should be given about who to call in a
crisis.

CONFUSIONAL STATES

The ability of the family to cope with a death in the home depends in
large measure on the doctor's ability to help both patient and family

to understand and cope with the confusional symptoms that ultimately occur in most cases. Sometimes, any sort of strange behaviour or talk in an ill patient is labelled 'confusion'. Unfortunately, once a patient is said to be confused, doctors, nurses, friends and family all tend to shy away in embarrassment, and sometimes in fear. Precision in assessment is necessary to enable the family and care givers to continue to respond appropriately to the patient who happens to be very ill and experiencing what is often only a minor disturbance of thought.

Similarly, a lack of discrimination can lead to nightmares, disorientation and momentary extensions of dreams into wakefulness being labelled as hallucinations. To call these common, normal phenomena 'hallucinations' can provoke anxiety because of the fear surrounding the word itself and the common assumption that their occurrence is synonymous with madness. On the other hand, the content of a patient's dreams may provide a useful window into the subconscious, and indicate fears about death that the patient has not yet been able to face up to at a conscious level.

If the 'hallucinations' are in fact just misperceptions, explanation by the doctor is often all that is necessary by way of treatment. However, when these phenomena are clearly expressions of anxiety about dying and death, anxiolytic medication may be helpful, together with continuing discussion about the experiences and possible psychological precipitating factors. Therapy with chlorpromazine – a common medical response to this situation – may help to suppress hallucinations but it may also increase the tendency to misperceive by causing further clouding of the sensorium.

A *confusional state* is characterized by 'clouding of the sensorium', and is usually associated with drowsiness. It manifests as one or more of the following:

(1)   Poor concentration,

(2)   Impairment of recent memory,

(3)   Disorientation,

(4)   Misperceptions (often) ± paranoid delusions,

(5)   Hallucinations (sometimes),

(6)   Rambling and incoherent speech,

(7)   Restlessness ± noisy/aggressive behaviour.

Confusional states tend to be variable in degree and intensity; in the dying most are caused by multiple factors. In some, the symptoms are never more than mild and remain intermittent. Those associated with metabolic disturbances (renal failure, hepatic failure, intestinal obstruction) tend to be more prolonged and more marked than those associated with terminal pneumonia which by definition is self-limiting.

Disorientation for time and, to a lesser extent, for place, is eventually quite normal in the dying. Explanation and reassurance may be all that is necessary, for example:

'When someone is not well, the mind often works more slowly, and doesn't always manage to stay in gear'.

'Most patients are like you – they lose track of time. After all, when you are not up and about and working, time is not so important, is it?'

Misperceptions are common too. A similar type of explanation is generally all that is necessary:

'It is something we all do at times, but, when you are ill, it tends to happen more often.'

'You are not losing your mind/going mad; this sort of thing can happen to any of us when we are very ill.'

AS DEATH APPROACHES

When the patient becomes increasingly weak he is faced with the fact that death is inevitable and imminent. This is the time when support and companionship are of paramount importance. Weakness is commonly associated with increasing somnolence or the need to rest for more prolonged periods during the day. Explanation is essential, for example:

'When the body is short of energy it takes a lot more effort to do even simple jobs. This means that you will need to rest more in order to restock your limited energy supply.'

For the patient who has not yet come to terms with the situation, the deterioration should be signalled gently, for example:

'I think a few quiet days in bed are called for. If tomorrow or the next day you are feeling more energetic, of course you should get up but, for the moment, bed is the best place for you.'

For the spouse and close family the explanation could be:

'This weakness is quite normal as his body is using all its energy to fight the tumour, but I think the illness is beginning to win.'

In the face of rapidly approaching death, the patient is often realistic. He knows you cannot perform a miracle, he appreciates that his time has come and, provided he is relatively comfortable, your continued attentiveness is all he expects of you. Although you feel powerless, the situation need never become totally negative and hopeless provided that you continue to visit and quietly indicate that 'at this stage the important thing is to keep you as comfortable as possible.'

Medication should be simplified as much as possible and should be given by suppository or injection when the patient is too weak to swallow. Steps should be taken to control an agitated delirium even if it results in greater somnolence. The family should be kept closely informed of the changing situation, for example:

'He is very weak now, but could still go on for several days.'

Finally, listen to the nurses who, particularly in hospital, are in continuing close contact with the patient when they are available.

Recommended reading

1. Saunders, C. (ed.) (1985). *The Management of Terminal Disease*, 2nd Edn. (London: Arnold)
2. Twycross, R. G. and Lack, S. A. (1984). *Therapeutics in Terminal Cancer*. (London: Pitman)
3. *Cancer Pain Relief*. (1986) (Geneva: WHO)

Appendix – Preparation of Solutions

PREPARATION OF NEUROLYTIC SOLUTIONS – PHENOL (HYDROXYBENZENE)

At 20°C one part phenol dissolves in 12 parts of water. Accordingly, phenol may be prepared in aqueous solution only in lower concentrations. If a stronger preparation is required a water–glycerin mixture is used as the solvent.

Product: phenol injection 5% in glycerin

Formula: phenol crystals 5 g
glycerin (previously dried at 120°C and cooled) to 100 g

Method of preparation: Dissolve the phenol in glycerin with the aid of gentle heat. Whilst still warm pass through a No. 3 sintered glass filter.

Packaging: Pack in 2 ml or 5 ml ampoules. Protect from light. Store in a cool place.

Sterilization: Dry heat at 150°C for 1 h.

Stability: 1 year from date of manufacture.

Product: aqueous phenol 5%   phenol injection 7%

Formula: phenol crystals 5 g   phenol crystals 7 g
   water for injections   glycerin 50% v/v in water for injec-
   to 100 ml   tions to 100 ml

Method of preparation: Pass through sintered glass filter, pack in ampoules and sterilize by autoclaving at 115°C for 30 min.

Packaging: 2 ml or 5 ml ampoules. Protect from light. Store in a cool place.

Precautions: Avoid prolonged contact with rubber or plastics.

Stability: 1 year from date of sterilization.

INJECTION ABSOLUTE ALCOHOL

Method of preparation: In order to avoid absorption of moisture, the infiltration procedure is best carried out under positive pressure, using solvent inert membrane filters. The preparation is then packed in 2 ml or 5 ml ampoules.

Sterilization: Autoclave at 155°C for 30 min.

Special precautions: Absolute alcohol absorbs moisture from the atmosphere: once the ampoule is opened the content should be used at once.

Stability: 2 years from date of sterilization.

PREPARATION OF ORAL MORPHINE SOLUTION

Product: oral morphine 5% (1 ml = 5 g)

Formula: Morphine hydrochloride or sulphate powder 5 g
   + disodium edetate 50 mg
   sodium metabisulphite 1 g
   benzoic acid 1 g or
   + distilled water to 1 L

   Amber glass bottles

   Shelf life: 6 months

Method of preparation: Dissolve powder in fresh distilled water. Add preservative (chloroform water or benzoic acid or alcohol) to 1000 ml.

Packaging: 100 ml bottle. (1 ml will contain 5 mg). Protect from light. Store in a cool place.

Stability: Up to 6 weeks.

PREPARATION OF EPIDURAL MORPHINE

Product: Epidural morphine

Formula: 1 cg/1 ml vial of morphine sulphate

Preparation: Dissolve in 9 ml distilled water in a sterile 10 ml syringe

SALIVA REPLACEMENT SOLUTION

Syrup 40 ml
Glycerin to 200 ml

Shelf life: 1 month

Glossary

Afferent   A nerve fibre carrying stimuli from the periphery to the central nervous system

Algesic   Pain causing

Algogenic   Pain producing

Allocheiria   Reference of pain to the opposite side of the body

Allodynia   Pain (such as referred pain) which occurs on non-noxious stimulation of normal skin

Analgesia   Absence of pain on noxious stimulation

Antidromic   Impulse transmitted opposite to the normal direction

Causalgia   A syndrome which follows a traumatic nerve lesion, comprising burning pain, vasomotor and sudomotor dysfunction and eventually trophic changes

Central pain   Pain caused by a lesion in the CNS

Commissure   A band of nerve fibres which run across the midline of the cord connecting corresponding parts on each side

Deafferentation   Nerve cells disconnected from normal afferent input

Decubitus   From the posture or position when lying in bed

Denervated   Deprived of innervation

Dysaesthesia   Unpleasant, abnormal sensation

Efferent   A nerve fibre carrying stimuli from the CNS to the periphery

Endorphinergic   Nerve fibres which release endorphin

Enkephalinergic   Nerve fibres which release enkephalin
Hyperaesthesia   Great sensitivity to any somatic stimulation
Hyperalgesia   Increased sensitivity to noxious stimulation
Hyperpathia   A painful response to a stimulus involving delayed
    reaction, over-reaction and after-sensation
Hypoaesthesia   Diminished sensitivity to any somatic stimulation
Hypoalgesia   Diminished sensitivity to noxious stimulation
Hypotonia   Reduced muscle tone
Inhibition   A restraining effect
Lancinating   Intermittent, sharp shooting or stabbing (pain)
Nociceptor   Nerve receptor which responds to painful stimuli
Noxious   Pain causing
Opioids   Narcotic analgesics
Paraesthesia   A 'pins and needles' type of disturbance of sensation
Somatotopical   Orderly representation of part of the body in a part
    of the CNS
Synapse   Junction between two nerve cells

Index

From the World Health Organization

CANCER PAIN RELIEF

*A book that promises to make pain relief
a routine component of cancer care*

In a concise, didactic, and logical way, *Cancer Pain Relief* sets forth information and arguments designed to correct the many false assumptions and faulty practices that hinder the relief of pain in cancer patients. Coverage ranges from statistics on the number of cancer patients who suffer unrelieved pain each day, through reasons for the inadequate use of established and highly effective treatments, to details on a method of treatment capable of relieving pain in 80–90% of patients. Throughout the book, emphasis is placed on the central importance of analgesic drugs and the need for guidance in their use.

The book has two main parts. The first provides background information on the prevalence and nature of cancer pain, the reasons for its inadequate control, and the steps necessary for improvement on a global scale. Basic principles of management are outlined and the need for professional and public education is discussed.

The second part of the book presents a detailed yet simple method of pain relief based on the sequential use of aspirin, codeine, and morphine administered 'by the clock'. This 'three-step ladder' method, which was worked out and agreed upon by more than 40 experts, shows how the correct use of a small number of safe, effective, and inexpensive drugs can provide complete and continuous pain relief in the vast majority of patients.

For doctors and nurses who lack formal training in pain management, *Cancer Pain Relief* will be welcomed as a source of sound, practical advice certain to improve their competence when working with cancer patients. The book should also be read by all public health authorities and hospital managers seeking to implement comprehensive programmes for the relief of cancer pain.

Cancer Pain Relief
World Health Organization, 1986
74 pages; available in English or French
ISBN: 92-4-156100-9
Sw.fr. 13.–/US$7.80

Available from:
World Health Organization
Distribution and Sales
1211 Geneva 27
Switzerland